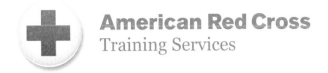

American Red Cross
Training Services

American Red Cross

CPR/AED for Professional Rescuers

Participant's Handbook

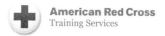
American Red Cross
Training Services

This Participant's Manual is part of the American Red Cross CPR/AED for Professional Rescuers program. The emergency care procedures outlined in the program materials reflect the standard of knowledge and accepted emergency practices in the United States at the time this manual was published. It is the reader's responsibility to stay informed of changes in emergency care procedures.

SCIENCE AND TECHNICAL CONTENT

The scientific content and evidence within the American Red Cross CPR/AED for Professional Rescuers program is consistent with the American Red Cross Aquatic Guidelines and Best Practices and the most current science and treatment recommendations from:

+ The International Liaison Committee on Resuscitation (ILCOR)

+ The International Federation of Red Cross and Red Crescent Societies

+ The Policy Statements, Evidence Reviews and Guidelines of:

  − American Academy of Pediatrics (AAP)

  − American College of Emergency Physicians (ACEP)

  − American College of Obstetrics and Gynecology (ACOG)

  − American College of Surgeons (ACS)

  − Committee on Tactical Combat Casualty Care (CoTCCC)

  − Obstetric Life Support™ (OBLS™)

  − Society of Critical Care Medicine (SCCM) and the American College of Critical Care Medicine (ACCM)

  − Surviving Sepsis Campaign (SSC)

Guidance for this course was provided by the American Red Cross Scientific Advisory Council, a panel of 60+ nationally and internationally recognized experts from a variety of medical, nursing, EMS, advanced practice, allied health, scientific, educational and academic disciplines. Members of the Scientific Advisory Council have a broad range of professional specialties including resuscitation, emergency medicine, critical care, obstetrics, pediatrics, anesthesia, cardiology, surgery, trauma, toxicology, pharmacology, education, sports medicine, occupational health, public health and emergency preparedness. This gives the Scientific Advisory Council the important advantage of broad, multidisciplinary expertise in evaluating existing and new assessment methodologies, technologies, therapies and procedures—and the educational methods to teach them.

More information on the science of the course content can be found at the following websites:

+ ilcor.org

+ redcross.org/science

ACKNOWLEDGMENTS

Many individuals were involved in the development and revision process in various supportive, technical and creative ways. The American Red Cross CPR/AED for Professional Rescuers Handbook was developed through the dedication of employees and volunteers. Their commitment to excellence made this handbook possible.

TABLE OF CONTENTS

SKILL SHEETS

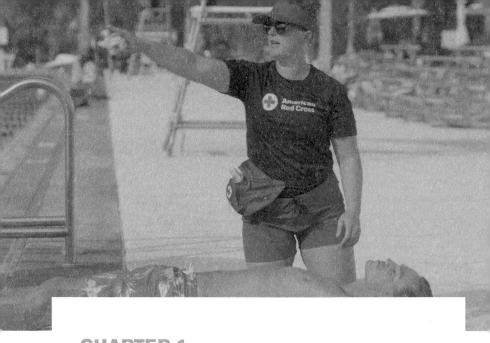

CHAPTER 1
FOUNDATIONAL CONCEPTS

As a professional rescuer, you have a duty to provide emergency care until more advanced emergency medical services (EMS) professionals take over. As a rescuer trained at the professional level, your major responsibilities are to ensure safety for yourself and others in the area, identify any immediate threats to the person's life, ensure that EMS has been called (as needed) and provide care consistent with your level of training until EMS professionals arrive and take over.

1:1 THE EMERGENCY MEDICAL SERVICES SYSTEM

The **emergency medical services (EMS) system** is a network of professionals linked together to provide the best care for people in all types of emergencies. Activating the EMS system occurs when someone recognizes an emergency and decides to take action by calling 9-1-1 or the designated emergency number. The emergency dispatcher obtains information about the emergency and provides this information to trained EMS professionals who respond to the scene. EMS professionals have advanced training that allows them to provide medical care outside of a hospital setting. Once on the scene, EMS professionals take over care of the person, including transportation to a hospital or other facility if necessary.

As a professional rescuer, you are an important link in the EMS system. Your role in the EMS system includes:

+ Recognizing that an emergency exists.

+ Taking action, including assessing the scene and the person, activating the EMS system and giving care until EMS professionals arrive and begin their care of the person.

To optimize functioning of the EMS system and increase the injured or ill person's chances for survival and recovery, every person who is involved with recognizing and responding to an emergency must perform their role promptly and correctly.

1:2 LEGAL PRINCIPLES THAT APPLY TO PROFESSIONAL RESCUERS

As a professional rescuer, there are certain expectations and standards for how you do your job. Failing to meet these expectations and standards can lead to legal action being taken against you, your employer, or both. Legal principles that apply to your role as a professional rescuer include the following.

Duty to Act

While on the job, you have a legal responsibility to act when an emergency occurs at your facility. Failure to act in an emergency could result in legal action.

Standard of Care

The standard of care establishes minimum expectations for professional rescuers in fulfilling their primary job responsibility, which is to prevent and respond to emergencies. The standard of care may be established in part by your training program and in part by state or local authorities. The standard of care requires you to:

+ Communicate proper information and warnings to help prevent injuries.

+ Recognize someone in need of care.

+ Provide emergency care according to your level of training.

Negligence

Negligence is failure to do what a reasonable and careful person would be expected to do in a given situation. When a person is injured or suffers additional harm because a professional rescuer failed to follow the standard of care or failed to act at all, the professional rescuer may be considered negligent. Examples of negligence include:

+ Failing to control or stop any behaviors that could result in further harm or injury.

+ Failing to provide care or providing inappropriate care.

+ Providing care outside of your **scope of practice** (the range of tasks you are legally allowed to do) or level of training.

INFO TO KNOW

The majority of states and the District of Columbia have Good Samaritan laws in place to help protect people who voluntarily give care in good faith without accepting or expecting anything in return. Some Good Samaritan laws, however, do not provide coverage for people who have a legal duty to act. If you have questions regarding whether or not you are protected when providing first aid, refer to your state's Good Samaritan laws.

Abandonment

Abandonment is withdrawal of support or help from another person, despite having the responsibility to provide this support or help. Once you begin providing care, you must continue to provide care until emergency medical services (EMS) professionals or someone with equal or greater training takes over. Leaving the scene or stopping care too soon would be considered examples of abandonment.

Confidentiality

You are required by law to keep any personal information that you learn about a person while providing care (for example, information about medical conditions, injuries or treatment) confidential. Do not share this information with anyone except EMS professionals directly involved in the person's care, your management team or your employer's legal counsel. Sharing personal information with individuals who are not directly involved with the person's medical care (such as reporters, insurance investigators or outside legal counsel) may be considered a violation of the person's right to privacy and confidentiality. If someone asks you for information and you are not sure whether you should share this information, refer the person to your manager.

Consent

A person must give **consent**, or permission, before you can provide first aid and emergency care. To obtain consent, tell the person your name, the type and level of training that you have and what you plan to do. With this information, the person can give you their consent for care or state that they do not wish for you to do anything. A person who appears unresponsive or mentally altered (for example, confused or disoriented) may not be able to give consent. In these cases, the law assumes the person would give consent if they could. This is called **implied consent**. Implied consent also applies when a minor (a person younger than 18 years in most states) needs emergency medical assistance and the minor's parent or guardian is not present. If the minor's parent or guardian is present, you should obtain their consent regardless of the minor's **level of consciousness** (state of awareness, alertness and wakefulness).

Refusal of Care

A person may refuse care (that is, not give consent for you to provide first aid or emergency care). A parent or guardian may also refuse care on behalf of a minor. When a person refuses care, you must honor their wishes. However, you should explain why you think care is necessary. If the person refuses care and the person's injury or illness is not life-threatening, make it clear that you are not denying or withholding care and that you are not abandoning the person. If you believe the person is seriously injured or experiencing a life-threatening medical emergency, call EMS professionals to evaluate the situation, but do not provide care.

1:3 LOWERING THE RISK FOR DISEASE TRANSMISSION

When you are working as a professional rescuer, you may be exposed to blood, body fluids or other potentially infectious materials that could contain pathogens. Being knowledgeable about how pathogens are spread, taking standard precautions and following your employer's infection control policies and procedures will help you to protect yourself and others from infectious disease.

The Body's Natural Defenses

The body has many natural defenses against infection. Healthy, intact skin and mucous membranes help to prevent microorganisms from entering the body. Reflexes, such as coughing and sneezing, help to expel microorganisms from the body. Finally, if a pathogen does gain access to the body, the immune system works to fight off the infection. Even though our bodies have ways of protecting us from infection and there are medications available to treat some infections, prevention is still the optimal goal.

Taking good care of your physical health, such as by getting adequate sleep and exercise, following a healthy diet and keeping your immunizations up to date, lowers your susceptibility to infection and helps to prevent the spread of infection to others.

The Chain of Infection

For infection to occur, six requirements must be met. These six requirements are the links in the chain of infection (Figure 1-1). Eliminating just one link in the chain can prevent an infection from spreading.

1. **Pathogen.** For an infection to occur, a microorganism that can cause disease must be present.

2. **Reservoir.** The pathogen must have a place to grow and multiply so that it is present in sufficient quantity to cause disease. Possible reservoirs include the bodies of people and animals, bodies of water and food.

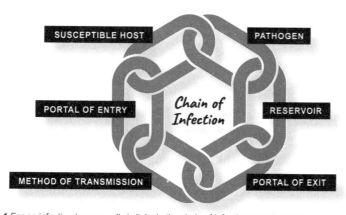

Figure 1-1 For an infection to occur, all six links in the chain of infection must be present.

3. **Portal of exit.** The pathogen must have a way of leaving the reservoir. The portal of exit varies depending on the pathogen and the reservoir. When the reservoir is the human body, the portal of exit may be the respiratory tract, the digestive tract, the genitourinary tract or breaks in the skin.

4. **Method of transmission.** The way a pathogen gets from one person to another is its method of transmission. The method of transmission may be direct or indirect (Figure 1-2). **Direct transmission** occurs when a pathogen is passed from one person to another through physical contact or droplet spread. **Indirect transmission** occurs when pathogens are spread by way of a contaminated surface or object or by a **vector** (an insect or animal, such as a mosquito, tick or rodent, that carries and transmits the pathogen).

5. **Portal of entry.** The pathogen must have a way of gaining entry to a new reservoir. Potential portals of entry include the respiratory tract, the digestive tract, the genitourinary tract, the eye and breaks in the skin.

6. **Susceptible host.** Finally, the pathogen must enter a susceptible host, or a person who is capable of becoming infected with that particular pathogen.

Standard Precautions

Standard precautions are safety measures you should take with every person to protect yourself and others from pathogens that are transmitted

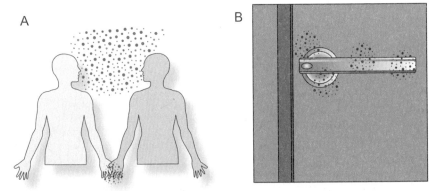

Figure 1-2 (A) In direct transmission, the pathogen is passed from one person to another through direct or close physical contact between two people or with droplets. **(B)** In indirect transmission, the pathogen is passed from one person to another via a contaminated object or a vector.

in blood, body fluids or other potentially infectious materials. Anyone's blood or body fluids might contain pathogens, even if the person appears to be healthy. For this reason, you should follow standard precautions every time you give care.

Hand Hygiene

Cleaning your hands properly and at the right times is the most important way to protect yourself and others from infection (Figure 1-3). At minimum, wash your hands:

+ Before giving care (if time allows).

+ After providing care, even if you wore gloves.

+ After touching blood, body fluids or other potentially infectious materials.

+ After touching objects or surfaces that could be contaminated with blood, body fluids or other potentially infectious materials.

+ Before putting on and after removing gloves or other personal protective equipment.

+ Before and after eating and drinking.

+ After using the restroom.

Wash your hands using soap and water for at least 20 seconds. Make sure to cover all surfaces of both hands: the palms and backs of your hands, in between your fingers (including the sides of your thumbs) and under your fingernails.

If soap and water are not available, you can use an alcohol-based hand sanitizer to clean your hands. Dispense the recommended amount of product into the palm of one hand and rub your hands together to cover all surfaces of your hands and fingers. Continue rubbing your hands together until they are

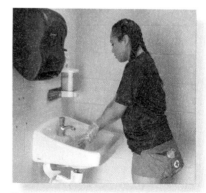

Figure 1-3 Washing your hands is essential to protect yourself and others from infection.

dry, which takes about 20 seconds. Although using an alcohol-based hand sanitizer properly will reduce the number of pathogens on your hands, it may not eliminate all pathogens, so always wash your hands with soap and water as soon as handwashing facilities are available.

Personal Protective Equipment

Personal protective equipment (PPE) is specialized equipment that is worn or used to prevent pathogens from contaminating your skin, mucous membranes or clothing (Figure 1-4). Examples of PPE include latex-free disposable gloves, resuscitation masks, bag-valve-mask (BVM) resuscitators, high-efficiency particulate air (HEPA) filter attachments, gowns, protective eyewear, face shields and face masks. PPE appropriate for your job duties should be available at your workplace.

Use PPE as indicated by the situation. For example, when there is a possibility that blood or other potentially infectious materials will splash or spray, wear a gown, face mask and protective eyewear in addition to gloves (Table 1-1).

Latex-free disposable gloves

Latex-free disposable gloves may be made of vinyl or nitrile. Nitrile latex-free disposable gloves are impermeable to blood, body fluids and other potentially infectious materials and should be worn when providing care.

Latex-free disposable gloves are meant to be worn once and then discarded. Never clean or reuse disposable gloves. Disposable gloves

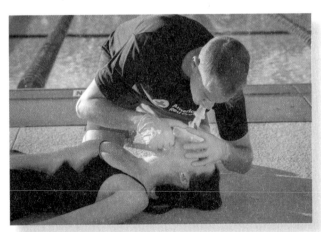

Figure 1-4 Always use personal protective equipment as appropriate for the situation and in accordance with your facility's exposure control plan.

Table 1-1 Recommended PPE for Protection from Bloodborne Pathogens in Prehospital Settings

Situation	Personal Protective Equipment			
	Disposable Gloves	Gown	Mask	Protective Eyewear
Bleeding control with spraying blood	Yes	Yes	Yes	Yes
Bleeding control with minimal bleeding	Yes	No	No	No
Emergency childbirth	Yes	Yes	Yes	Yes
Oral or nasal suctioning of the airway, manually clearing airway	Yes	No, unless soiling is likely	Yes	Yes
Handling and cleaning equipment and clothing contaminated with blood	Yes	No, unless soiling is likely	No	No

should fit properly and be free of rips or tears. Wear latex-free disposable gloves:

+ When providing care, especially whenever there is a possibility that you will come in contact with a person's blood, body fluids or other potentially infectious materials.

+ When there is a break in the skin on your own hands. (Cover any cuts, scrapes or sores before putting on the gloves.)

+ When you must handle items or surfaces soiled with blood, body fluids or other potentially infectious materials.

When you are wearing gloves, try to limit how much you touch other surfaces with your gloved hands. Pathogens from your soiled gloves can transfer to other items or surfaces that you touch, putting the next person who handles the item or touches the surface at risk for infection. If possible, remove soiled gloves and replace them with a clean pair before touching other surfaces or equipment. When multiple people need care, remove your gloves, wash your hands, and replace your gloves with a clean pair before assisting the next person.

To remove your gloves, you must use proper technique to avoid contaminating your own skin (Skill Sheet 1-1). Dispose of the gloves properly. Your facility may have policies that define when gloves should be disposed of in a red biohazard waste bag. Then, wash your hands.

CPR breathing barriers

Always use a CPR breathing barrier, such as a resuscitation mask or BVM resuscitator, when giving ventilations. CPR breathing barriers cover the person's mouth and nose and protect you from contact with saliva and other body fluids, such as blood and vomit, as you give ventilations. Breathing barriers also protect you from breathing the air that the person exhales.

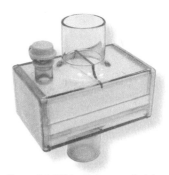

Figure 1-5 A high-efficiency particulate air (HEPA) filter attachment can be used with a bag-valve-mask resuscitator or a resuscitation mask to provide additional protection from pathogens in exhaled air.

A HEPA filter attachment (Figure 1-5) can be used with a BVM resuscitator or a resuscitation mask. The HEPA filter traps viruses, bacteria and other microorganisms in exhaled air to provide additional protection from pathogens while you are giving ventilations. The bacterial and viral filtration efficiency is greater than 99.99%. To be effective, the HEPA filter must be kept dry.

Cleaning and Disinfection

Reusable equipment and surfaces that have been contaminated by blood, body fluids or other potentially infectious materials need to be properly cleaned and disinfected before the equipment is put back into service or the area is reopened (Box 1-1).

Box 1-1 CLEANING AND DISINFECTING SURFACES AND EQUIPMENT

Clean and disinfect equipment and surfaces that have been soiled with blood, body fluids or other potentially infectious materials as soon as possible after the incident occurs. Remember to wear appropriate personal protective equipment (PPE).

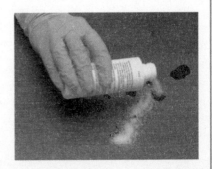

Continued

Box 1-1 CLEANING AND DISINFECTING SURFACES AND EQUIPMENT (Continued)

+ Prevent others from accessing the area or using the equipment.

+ If the spill contains a sharp object (for example, shards of broken glass), use tongs or a disposable scoop and scraper to remove and dispose of the object. Never pick the object up with your hands.

+ Clean and disinfect the equipment or surface according to your facility's protocols.

If there is no protocol, follow this general approach for cleaning and disinfecting equipment and surfaces:

1. Wipe up or absorb the spill using absorbent wipes or a solidifier (a fluid-absorbing powder).

2. Remove your disposable latex-free gloves, wash your hands, and put on a clean pair of gloves to protect yourself while using the disinfectant. When using a bleach solution as a disinfectant, always ensure good ventilation and wear gloves and eye protection.

3. Flood the area with a freshly mixed disinfectant solution of approximately 1½ cups of bleach and 1 gallon of water (1 part bleach to 9 parts water, or about a 10 percent solution) or use another approved disinfectant product.

4. Let the disinfectant stand on the surface for the recommended amount of time. If you are using a bleach solution, this is at least 10 minutes.

5. Use clean absorbent materials (such as paper towels) to wipe up the disinfectant and dry the area.

6. Dispose of all materials used to clean up the spill in a labeled biohazard container. If a biohazard container is not available, place the soiled materials in a sealable plastic bag or a plastic container with a lid, seal the bag or container, and dispose of it properly.

Bloodborne Pathogens and Workplace Safety

As a professional rescuer, you must take measures to protect yourself and others from *all* infections. However, some infections pose particular risk because of their potential to have long-term effects on your health if you become infected. Many of the most serious infections that professional rescuers may be exposed to on the job are caused by **bloodborne pathogens** (disease-causing microorganisms that are spread when blood from an infected person enters the bloodstream of a person who is not infected).

Although bloodborne pathogens can cause serious illnesses, they are not easily transmitted and are not spread by casual contact. For infection to occur, an infected person's blood must enter your bloodstream. This could happen through direct or indirect contact with an infected person's blood if it comes in contact with your eyes, the mucous membranes that line your mouth and nose, or an area of broken skin on your body. You could also become infected if you stick yourself with a contaminated needle (a "needlestick injury") or cut yourself with something that has been soiled with blood.

Bloodborne pathogens that can cause serious infections include hepatitis B virus (HBV), hepatitis C virus (HCV) and human immunodeficiency virus (HIV) (Table 1-2).

+ Hepatitis is inflammation of the liver, an organ that performs many vital functions for the body. Chronic infection with the viruses that cause hepatitis B or C can lead to liver failure, liver cancer and other serious conditions. A vaccine is available to protect against HBV. However, there is no vaccine to protect against HCV.

+ HIV is a virus that attacks white blood cells and destroys the body's ability to fight infection. Over time, people infected with HIV may develop acquired immunodeficiency syndrome (AIDS), which is the most advanced stage of HIV infection. A person with AIDS has a very impaired immune system. As a result, they get an increasing number of severe illnesses, called opportunistic infections. Although there are medications that can help slow the progression of HIV infection, currently there is no cure for AIDS and no vaccine to protect against HIV infection.

Use of PPE, such as gloves, is an important method of protecting yourself from exposure to bloodborne pathogens. You should put gloves on as soon as time permits in situations involving possible contact with blood, body fluids or other potentially infectious materials; mucous membranes; or non-intact

Table 1-2 Bloodborne Pathogens of Primary Concern to Professional Rescuers

Pathogen	Signs and Symptoms of Acute Infection	Long-Term Consequences of Infection	Mode of Transmission	Infectious Material	Risk for Infection Following Needlestick or Cut Exposure
Hepatitis B virus (HBV)	Fever, fatigue, loss of appetite, nausea, vomiting, abdominal pain, dark urine, clay-colored stool, joint pain, jaundice (yellow color of the skin and eyes)	Liver damage, liver failure, liver cancer, death	• Direct contact • Indirect contact	Blood, saliva, vomit, semen	**Vaccinated:** virtually no risk **Unvaccinated:** as high as 30%
Hepatitis C virus (HCV)	Fever, fatigue, dark urine, clay-colored stool, abdominal pain, loss of appetite, nausea, vomiting, joint pain, jaundice (yellow color of the skin and eyes)	Mild to severe chronic liver disease, cirrhosis (scarring of the liver), liver cancer, need for liver transplant	• Direct contact • Indirect contact	Blood, saliva, vomit, semen	About 2%
Human immuno-deficiency virus (HIV)	Fever, chills, rash, night sweats, muscle aches, sore throat, fatigue, swollen lymph nodes, mouth ulcers; some people have no signs or symptoms	Opportunistic infections (for example, severe pneumonia, tuberculosis), cancers, death	• Direct contact • Possibly indirect contact	Blood, semen, vaginal fluid, breast milk	Less than 1%

skin. However, do not delay providing potentially lifesaving care to put on gloves. Your risk for infection from HIV and other bloodborne pathogens is very low. The risk for contracting HIV as a result of infected blood coming into contact with non-intact skin is less than 0.1%. There is no risk for contracting HIV if infected blood comes into contact with intact skin. Always know and follow your employer's guidelines for what PPE to use and when.

OSHA Bloodborne Pathogens Standard

You and your employer share the responsibility for protecting you from **occupational exposure** to bloodborne pathogens (contact with blood, body fluids or other potentially infectious materials that may occur while you are performing your job duties). To effectively limit your risk for exposure to bloodborne pathogens while you are on the job, you must practice standard precautions consistently and correctly. Your employer must make sure you have the training and equipment you need to lower your risk. Standards that employers must follow to keep their employees safe from occupational exposures to bloodborne pathogens are outlined in the **Occupational Safety and Health Administration (OSHA) Bloodborne Pathogens Standard** (Box 1-2).

Box 1-2 OSHA BLOODBORNE PATHOGENS STANDARD

To protect employees from exposure on the job to bloodborne pathogens, employers are required to adhere to the following standards:

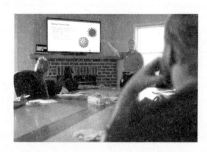

+ **Exposure control plan.** The facility must have a written plan that outlines actions that will be taken to eliminate or minimize employees' risk of exposure to blood or other potentially infectious materials on the job. The plan must be reviewed at least annually and made available in written form to all employees with an occupational risk for exposure to

Continued

Box 1-2 OSHA BLOODBORNE PATHOGENS STANDARD (Continued)

bloodborne pathogens. Employees are responsible for reporting exposure incidents so that proper follow-up (for example, medical testing) can be provided.

+ **Training.** Employers must provide training to all employees who may be exposed to bloodborne pathogens on the job about risks associated with bloodborne pathogens and how to minimize these risks. Training should be provided at the employee orientation and then at regular intervals thereafter.

+ **Personal protective equipment.** Employers are responsible for providing personal protective equipment (PPE) for employee use.

+ **HBV vaccination.** Employers must offer employees who have a risk of exposure to blood or other potentially infectious materials an opportunity to receive at no cost a vaccination that protects against hepatitis B. The vaccination must be made available within 10 working days of assignment to a job where there is a risk for occupational exposure, after appropriate training has been completed. If an employee decides not to be vaccinated, the employee must sign a form affirming the decision.

+ **Work practice controls.** The employer is responsible for establishing and enforcing policies and procedures that reduce the likelihood of an exposure incident and for supplying the equipment needed to follow these policies and procedures. Examples of work practice controls include requiring employees to wear PPE when performing certain job duties, establishing procedures for the disposal of contaminated materials, establishing procedures for cleaning and disinfecting equipment and surfaces, and establishing protocols for when hands should be washed.

+ **Engineering controls.** The employer is responsible for making equipment available that employees can use to protect themselves and others from exposure, such as PPE, sharps disposal containers, and biohazard bags and labels.

Handling an Exposure Incident

If another person's blood, body fluids or other potentially infectious material comes into contact with your eyes, the mucous membranes of your mouth or nose, or an opening or break in your skin, or if you experience a needlestick injury or cut yourself with something that has been soiled with blood, then you have been involved in an exposure incident. If an exposure incident occurs:

+ Immediately take steps to decontaminate the site of the exposure. If your skin was exposed, wash the area with soap and water. For splashes into your mouth or nose, flush the area with water. For splashes into your eyes, irrigate them with water, saline or a sterile irrigating solution for 15 to 20 minutes.

+ Follow your employer's exposure control plan for reporting the incident and receiving post-exposure follow-up care. You should notify the appropriate people at your place of employment about the incident and seek immediate follow-up care according to your employer's exposure control plan. You must also complete any necessary documentation according to the exposure control plan. Document the time and date of the exposure, the circumstances of the exposure, the actions taken after the exposure and other relevant information about the incident.

1:4 WRAP-UP

As a professional rescuer, you are an important link in the emergency medical services (EMS) system. When an emergency occurs, you have a duty to act and to provide emergency care according to your level of training. When providing emergency care, you must take appropriate precautions to protect yourself and others from the transmission of infectious diseases.

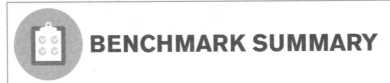

BENCHMARK SUMMARY

Benchmarks for Professional Rescuers

Professional rescuers should:

+ Expect to be equipped with and ready to use personal protective equipment (PPE).

+ Obtain consent, identifying themselves as trained rescuers.

1	Pinch the palm side of one glove on the outside near your wrist.	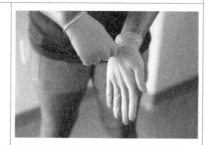
2	Pull the glove toward your fingertips, turning it inside out as you pull it off your hand.	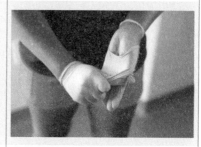
3	Hold the glove in the palm of your other (still-gloved) hand.	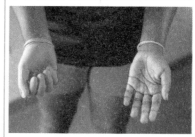
4	Carefully slip two fingers under the wrist of the other glove. • Avoid touching the outside of the glove.	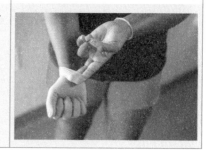

Continued

Skill Sheet 1-1. **Removing Disposable Gloves (Continued)**

5 Pull the glove toward your fingertips, turning it inside out as you pull it off your hand. The other glove is now contained inside.

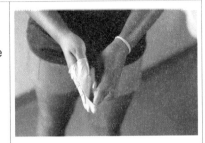

6 Dispose of the gloves properly and wash your hands.

• Follow your facility's policies for when gloves should be disposed of in a red biohazard waste bag.

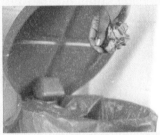

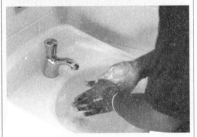

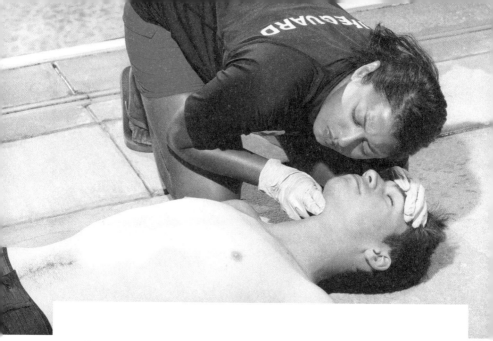

CHAPTER 2
ASSESSMENT

As a rescuer trained at the professional level, your major responsibilities are to ensure safety for yourself and others in the area, identify any immediate threats to the person's life, ensure that EMS has been called (as needed) and provide care consistent with your level of training until EMS professionals arrive and take over. **Assessment** is the process of gathering data about the emergency and the person that helps you to determine appropriate next actions. To ensure that the most critical problems are addressed first, take a systematic approach to assessment. Perform a rapid assessment and, when the person's condition allows, a secondary assessment.

2:1 RAPID ASSESSMENT

The information you gather during the rapid assessment helps you to ensure your own safety and the safety of others in the area and to recognize life-threatening conditions that need to be addressed right away. The rapid assessment (Figure 2-1) includes:

+ Performing a scene size-up, including checking the scene for safety and forming an initial impression of the person.

+ Checking for responsiveness.

+ Opening the airway and simultaneously checking for breathing, a pulse and life-threatening bleeding.

+ Giving 2 ventilations if appropriate.

+ Providing care based on the conditions found.

Perform a Scene Size-Up

During the scene size-up, you will:

+ Assess the scene to identify safety hazards, evaluate the number of injured or ill people and look for clues about what may have caused the emergency and the injury or illness (Box 2-1).

+ Form an initial impression of the person, including noting whether the person appears to have any life-threatening conditions, such as unresponsiveness or life-threatening bleeding.

+ Determine what additional resources may be needed.

In any emergency, you need to first make sure the environment is safe—for you, your team and anyone else there. When assessing for safety, ask yourself:

+ Are any immediate dangers present?

+ What guidance needs to be given to others who may be present?

RAPID ASSESSMENT

LG - 2023 Version

Perform scene size-up

Land Emergency
- Check scene for safety
- Activate EAP
- Form initial impression

Water Emergency
- Check scene for safety
- Activate EAP
- Rescue and form an initial impression
- Extricate immediately if person appears to be unresponsive and not breathing

Check for responsiveness
- Shout-tap-shout

Assess for life-threatening bleeding. If at any time the person has life-threatening bleeding, control it with any available resource (including a tourniquet or hemostatic dressing as appropriate).

Responsive? —YES

NO

- **Summon EMS**; get equipment
- **Check for breathing and a pulse** (≤ 10 seconds)
- At the same time, **scan the body for life-threatening bleeding**

- **Position** person as appropriate for condition
- Perform **secondary assessment** as person's condition allows
- Continue to **monitor** person's condition until EMS professionals arrive and begin their care

Breathing? —YES→

NO

- If not breathing as a result of drowning, give **2 initial ventilations**

Respiratory Arrest / Respiratory Failure ←YES— **Pulse?** —NO→ **Cardiac Arrest**

A

- Provide **ventilations**
  - ° **Adult:** 1 ventilation every **6 sec**
  - ° **Child/infant:** 1 ventilation every 2-3 sec
- Continue to **check breathing and pulse every 2 min**; if pulse becomes absent, **go to A**
- Perform **secondary assessment** as person's condition allows
- Continue to **monitor** person's condition until EMS professionals arrive and begin their care

- Start **CPR**
  - ° **Adult:** 30:2
  - ° **Child/infant:** 30:2 (single rescuer)
    15:2 (multiple rescuer)
- Use **AED** as soon as it is available
- Continue CPR until:
  - ° You see signs of ROSC
  - ° An AED is ready to analyze the heart rhythm
  - ° Other trained providers take over
  - ° You are too exhausted to continue
  - ° The situation becomes unsafe

American Red Cross
Training Services

Figure 2-1 To ensure the most life-threatening conditions are addressed first, take a systematic approach to assessment.

Box 2-1 SCENE SIZE-UP

During the scene size-up, first assess the scene to identify safety hazards, evaluate the number of people who need help, and look for clues about what may have caused the emergency and how the person(s) became ill or injured.

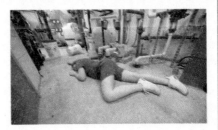

Safety

In any emergency, you must make sure the environment is safe for you and everyone else in the area. Use your senses to check for unusual odors, sights or sounds that could indicate danger, such as the smell of gas or smoke, a chemical spill on the ground or the sound of an alarm. If the scene appears to be unsafe, move to a safe distance, immediately call 9-1-1 or instruct someone to do so, and wait for medical, fire or police assistance to arrive. If you must leave the scene to ensure your own safety, you must make all attempts to move the person to safety as well. However, do not attempt to move the person if you cannot reach the person and remove them from the area without putting yourself in danger.

Number of Persons

It is important to note how many people are involved in the emergency. Take a complete 360-degree view of the area and ask others who are present whether anyone else was involved in the incident.

Nature of Illness or Mechanism of Injury

To determine the nature of the illness or the mechanism of injury, look for clues as to what may have caused the emergency and how the person became ill or injured—for example, the person's position or the presence of blood, broken glass or a spilled bottle of medication. Think critically about the situation and ask yourself

Continued

Box 2-1 SCENE SIZE-UP (Continued)

whether what you see makes sense. Quickly ask others who are present what happened and use the information to determine a likely cause. Keep in mind that a person may have moved or been moved before you arrived on the scene.

Next, form an initial impression about the person's condition and what is wrong. Your first impression is based entirely on the person's appearance. For example, does the person seem alert, or confused or sleepy? Look at the person's skin—does it appear to be its normal color, or does it seem pale, gray (ashen), blue (cyanotic) or flushed? Is the person moving, or motionless? Does the person have any immediately identifiable injuries? Pay particular attention to signs that the person may have a life-threatening condition. Ask yourself:

+ Does the person appear unresponsive?

+ Does the person seem to be breathing or are they having trouble breathing?

+ Is there life-threatening bleeding?

Then, quickly determine what additional resources are needed.

+ Who is available to help?

+ Do you need any additional equipment, such as an AED?

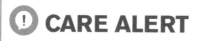

ⓘ CARE ALERT

If there is life-threatening bleeding, control it with any available resources (including the use of a tourniquet or hemostatic dressing as appropriate) and, if not already done, make sure EMS has been called.

Check for Responsiveness

Once the scene size-up is complete, the next step is to check for responsiveness. This may be obvious from your initial impression. For example, the person may be able to speak to you or they may be moaning, crying or moving around. If the person is responsive, obtain consent, complete a secondary assessment, and provide care as appropriate. If at any time life-threatening conditions develop or are found, stop your secondary assessment, instruct someone to call EMS and get emergency equipment, and give care for the condition according to your level of training.

 CARE ALERT

Remember that you must obtain consent from an awake and alert adult before you touch them to perform a secondary assessment or provide care. If the adult is not alert, consent is implied. For most infants and children up to the age of 18 years, you must obtain consent from the child's parent or legal guardian if they are present, regardless of the child's level of consciousness.

If the person appears unresponsive during the initial impression, check for responsiveness by using the **shout-tap-shout sequence** (Figure 2-2). First, shout "Are you OK?" using the person's name if you know it, then tap the person's shoulders (if the person is an adult or child) or the bottom of the person's foot (if the person is an infant) and shout again. If the person does not respond to you in any way—for example, by moving, opening their eyes or moaning—they are unresponsive. If you have not already done so, make sure EMS has been called and call for emergency equipment, including an AED.

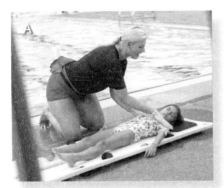 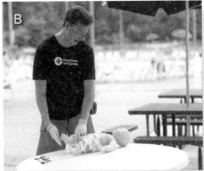

Figure 2-2 If the person appears unresponsive, check for responsiveness using the shout-tap-shout sequence. **(A)** In an adult or child, tap the shoulders. **(B)** In an infant, tap the bottom of the foot.

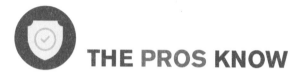

THE PROS KNOW

A person who can speak, cry or cough forcefully is responsive, has an open airway, is breathing and has a pulse.

Check for Breathing, a Pulse and Life-Threatening Bleeding

Next, if the person is unresponsive, simultaneously check for breathing, a pulse and life-threatening bleeding.

To check for breathing, you must open the person's airway (Figure 2-3). Make sure the person is in a supine (face-up) position. If they are face-down, roll them onto their back, taking care not to create or worsen a suspected injury. Then use one of the following techniques to open the airway:

+ **Head-tilt/chin-lift technique.** Position yourself at the person's side. Press down on the forehead with one hand while pulling up on the bony underside of the chin with two or three fingers of the other hand. Tilt the head back to a past-neutral position (for an adult), a slightly past-neutral position (for a child) or a neutral position (for an infant) as you lift up on the chin (Figure 2-4).

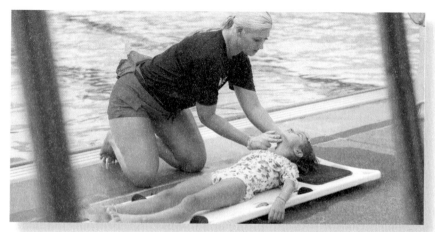

Figure 2-3 To check for breathing, you first need to open the airway.

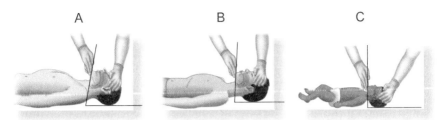

Figure 2-4 Tilt the person's head back to **(A)** the past-neutral position for an adult, **(B)** the slightly past-neutral position for a child and **(C)** the neutral position for an infant. In an infant, be careful not to tilt the head back too far because overextending the airway can block it.

+ **Jaw-thrust maneuver with head extension**. From above the person's head, put one hand on each side of the person's head with your thumbs near the corners of the mouth and pointed toward the chin. Slide your fingers under the angles of the jawbone. Thrust the jaw up and tilt the head back to a past-neutral position (for an adult), a slightly past-neutral position (for a child) or a neutral position (for an infant) to open the airway.

+ **Modified jaw-thrust maneuver.** Use a modified jaw-thrust maneuver when a person has a suspected head, neck or spinal injury. From above the person's head, put one hand on each side of the person's head, with your thumbs near the corners of the mouth and pointed toward the chin. Slide your fingers under the angles of the jawbone without moving the person's head or neck. Thrust the jaw up (again, without moving the head or neck) to lift the jaw and open the airway.

Skill Sheet 2-1 provides step-by-step instructions for opening the airway using these techniques.

Once the airway is open, simultaneously check for breathing and a pulse for **no more than 10 seconds** (Figure 2-5). Look again for life-threatening bleeding while checking for breathing and a pulse.

+ **To check for breathing:** Position your ear over the person's mouth and nose. Look to see if the person's chest is rising and falling, listen for escaping air and feel for breathing against the side of your cheek. Normal breathing is quiet, regular and effortless. **Agonal breaths** (isolated or infrequent gasps) are not normal breathing and are a sign

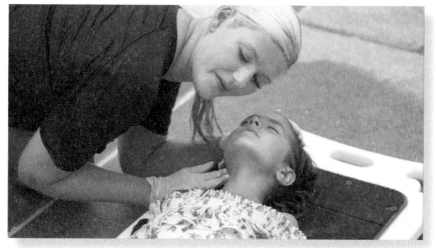

Figure 2-5 Simultaneously check for breathing and a pulse for no more than 10 seconds.

of cardiac arrest. If you observe agonal breaths, the person is not breathing.

+ **To check for a pulse:** In an adult or child, slide two fingers into the groove of the person's neck to feel for a carotid pulse (Figure 2-6A). In an infant, place two fingers on the inside of the upper arm between the elbow and the shoulder to feel for a brachial pulse (Figure 2-6B).

+ **To check for life-threatening bleeding:** While checking for breathing and a pulse, quickly scan down the body, looking for life-threatening bleeding that you may not have seen during the initial impression.

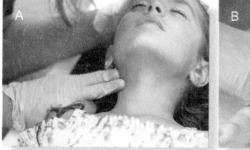
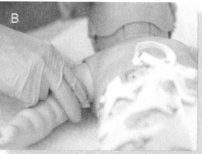

Figure 2-6 **(A)** In an adult or child, check for a carotid pulse. **(B)** In an infant, check for a brachial pulse.

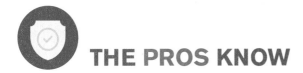

THE PROS KNOW

Use the A-B-C mnemonic to easily recall and perform the steps of the breathing and pulse check. Open the airway (A), check for the presence or absence of normal breathing (B) and simultaneously check for circulation (C) by a pulse check.

Give 2 Ventilations If Appropriate

A person who has been removed from the water and is not breathing is in immediate need of ventilations. Anyone who experiences respiratory impairment from submersion in water has drowned. Drowning may or may not result in death. In general, if a person is rescued quickly enough, giving ventilations may resuscitate them. Without oxygen, the person's heart will stop and death will result.

For a person who is not breathing as a result of drowning, give 2 ventilations as part of the rapid assessment before beginning care (Figure 2-7). Each ventilation should last about 1 second and make

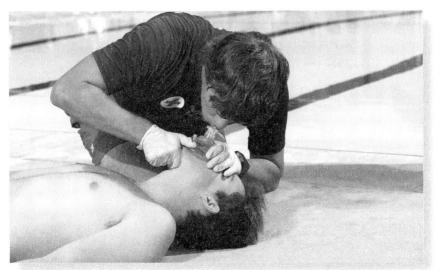

Figure 2-7 As part of the rapid assessment, give 2 ventilations to a person who is not breathing as a result of drowning.

the chest begin to rise. If the chest does not rise after either the first or the second ventilation, reopen the airway, make a seal, and try another ventilation for a total of 2 initial ventilations before beginning care. Do not attempt more than 3 ventilations before beginning care. You will learn how to give ventilations in Chapter 3.

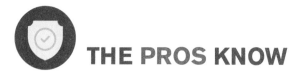

THE PROS KNOW

You may see a white or pinkish foam or froth coming out of the person's nose and mouth following a drowning. This is called **frothing** and it is caused by a mix of mucus, air and water during respiration. If you see frothing, complete your assessment, including providing 2 initial ventilations, and then begin care. Do not take time to wipe away the foam or froth.

Provide Care Based on the Conditions Found

The conditions that you find as a result of your rapid assessment determine your next actions.

Not Breathing, Pulse Present

If the person is unresponsive, is not breathing (or is breathing ineffectively) but has a pulse, the person is in **respiratory arrest** (breathing has stopped) or **respiratory failure** (the respiratory system is not able to meet the body's needs for oxygen delivery, carbon dioxide removal, or both). To care for respiratory arrest or respiratory failure, provide ventilations. You will learn how to care for respiratory arrest or respiratory failure in Chapter 3.

Not Breathing, No Pulse Present

If the person is unresponsive, is not breathing normally (or is only gasping) and has no pulse, the person is in **cardiac arrest** (the heart has stopped beating or is beating too ineffectively to circulate blood to the brain and other vital organs). The care for cardiac arrest is immediate CPR, starting with compressions, and use of an AED as soon as an AED is available. You will learn how to provide CPR and use an AED in Chapter 4.

Breathing and Pulse Present

If the person is breathing and has a pulse, position the person as appropriate for their condition, and perform the secondary assessment as the person's condition allows.

When a person is unresponsive but breathing or responsive but not fully awake, put them in a **recovery position** on their side if there are no obvious signs of a life-threatening injury or illness and if you do not suspect a head, neck or spinal injury (Figure 2-8, Box 2-2). The recovery position helps to lower the person's risk for choking and **aspiration** (inhalation of foreign matter, such as saliva or vomit, into the lungs). You should also use the recovery position if a person begins to vomit or if it is necessary to leave the person alone to summon EMS.

If you suspect a head, neck or spinal injury, leave the person in a face-up position unless you are unable to maintain an open airway because of fluids or vomit or if you have to leave the person alone to summon EMS.

Skill Sheet 2-2 provides step-by-step instructions for conducting a rapid assessment.

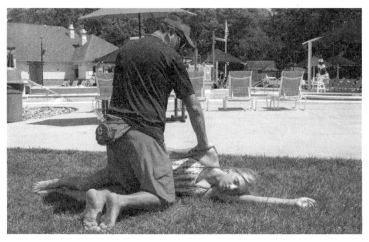

Figure 2-7 Use the recovery position if a person is unresponsive but breathing (or if they are responsive but not fully awake).

Box 2-2 RECOVERY POSITION

To place an adult, child or infant in the recovery position:

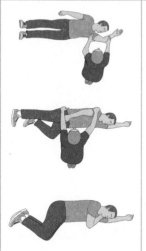

+ Extend the person's arm that is closest to you above the person's head.

+ Roll the person toward yourself onto their side, so that the person's head rests on their extended arm. Turning the person toward yourself, rather than away from yourself, allows for more control over the movement and helps you monitor the person's airway.

+ Bend both of the person's knees to stabilize their body.

2:2 SECONDARY ASSESSMENT

Perform a secondary assessment if the rapid assessment does not reveal any immediately life-threatening conditions. Remember, a person who is awake and alert must give consent before you assess them or give care.

The secondary assessment provides additional information about injuries or conditions that may require care and could become life-threatening if not addressed. The information that you gather during the secondary assessment will help you determine whether it is necessary to activate the EMS system (Box 2-3). If any life-threatening conditions develop or are found during your secondary assessment, immediately stop the assessment, instruct someone to call EMS and get emergency equipment, and give care for the condition according to your level of training. If necessary and additional rescuers are available, delegate care.

To conduct a secondary assessment, first obtain a focused history and then conduct a focused examination.

Box 2-3 WHEN TO ACTIVATE THE EMERGENCY MEDICAL SERVICES SYSTEM

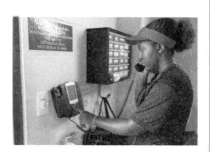

+ Unresponsiveness or an altered level of consciousness (LOC), such as drowsiness or confusion

+ Cardiac arrest (unresponsive; no breathing or only gasping; no pulse)

+ Choking (cannot cough, cry, speak or breathe; universal sign of choking)

+ Anaphylaxis (signs of allergic reaction; history of allergy; swelling of the face, neck, tongue or lips; trouble breathing; shock; change in responsiveness)

+ Breathing problems (trouble breathing or no breathing; asthma attack)

+ Chest pain, discomfort or pressure lasting more than a few minutes or that radiates to the shoulder, arm, neck, jaw, stomach or back

+ Persistent abdominal pain or pressure

+ Life-threatening external bleeding (bleeding that spurts or flows continuously from a wound or pools on surfaces; volume is about 6 ounces [¾ cup] or even less for small children and infants)

+ Vomiting blood or passing blood

+ Severe (critical) burns

+ Suspected poison exposure

+ Seizure in the water

+ Seizure on land under certain conditions (the person's first seizure, the seizure lasts more than 5 minutes or the person has multiple seizures in a row, the person was injured as a result of the seizure, the person is unresponsive and not breathing or only

Continued

Box 2-3 WHEN TO ACTIVATE THE EMERGENCY MEDICAL SERVICES SYSTEM (Continued)

gasping after the seizure, the person is pregnant, the person is known to have diabetes)

+ Signs or symptoms of stroke (drooping of the face on one side; sudden weakness on one side of the body; sudden slurred speech or difficulty speaking; sudden, severe headache)

+ Signs or symptoms of shock (changes in level of consciousness; rapid breathing; rapid, weak heartbeat; nausea or vomiting; pale, gray [ashen], cool, moist skin; restlessness or irritability; excessive thirst)

+ Opioid overdose (decreased breathing effort and rate; unresponsiveness; bluish or greyish skin color; small pupils)

+ Diabetic emergency (trouble breathing; fast or deep breathing; feeling weak or "different;" sweating; fast heartbeat)

+ Hypothermia (shivering; pale skin that is cold to the touch; disorientation)

+ Heat stroke (moist, pale or flushed skin; absence of sweating or some degree of sweating; unresponsiveness or confusion; seizure; headache; nausea; dizziness; weakness; exhaustion)

+ Suspected or obvious injuries to the head, neck or spine

+ Suspected or obvious broken bone

+ An injured or ill person who needs medical attention and cannot be moved

Focused History

Begin by asking the person's name and use it when you speak to them. Position yourself at eye level with the person and speak clearly, calmly and in a friendly manner, using age-appropriate language. Try to provide as much privacy as possible for the person while you are obtaining the history, and keep the history brief. Tailor your approach to the age of the person, as well as to any special circumstances.

Other people at the scene may be able to provide useful information as well. They may have witnessed what happened. If there are others at the scene who know the person well (such as family members or friends), they may be able to provide information about the person's medical history if the person is unable to do so (for example, because of the effects of illness or injury).

Use the SAMPLE mnemonic to guide your questions when obtaining the focused history.

+ **S = Signs and symptoms. Signs** are clues to the person's condition that you can observe for yourself, using one of your senses. For example, you may see that the person is sweating heavily, hear wheezing when the person is breathing, or feel that the person's skin is cool and moist. **Symptoms** are clues to the person's condition that only the person can describe to you, so you need to ask the person what they are feeling or experiencing. For example, the person may tell you that they are in pain, feeling nauseous, have a headache or feel dizzy. Ask follow-up questions as needed. For example, if the person reports pain, ask them where the pain is located, when the pain started and what the pain feels like (for example, "crushing," "stabbing," "throbbing").

+ **A = Allergies.** Ask the person if they are allergic to any foods, medications or things found in the environment (such as bees). If the person does report an allergy, ask what type of reaction the person had in the past when exposed to the allergen and what care the person received.

+ **M = Medications.** Ask the person if they are taking any prescription or over-the-counter medications. If the person is taking a medication, ask them what the medication is and whether they took it as prescribed today. Even if the person does not know the exact name or dose of the medication, they may still be able to tell you its purpose (for example, "I take blood pressure medication").

+ **P = Past medical history.** Ask the person whether they have any medical conditions; whether they have recently been ill; and whether they have recently had surgery, a medical emergency or been hospitalized.

+ **L = Last oral intake.** Ask when the person last had something to eat or drink.

+ **E = Events.** Ask the person what was happening and what they were doing just before they began to feel ill or became injured.

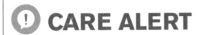

CARE ALERT

Remember that you are required by law to keep any personal information that you learn about a person confidential. Do not share this information with anyone except EMS professionals directly involved in the person's care, your management team or your employer's legal counsel.

Focused Examination

Next, complete a focused examination. Before beginning, tell the person what you are going to do. The idea of this check is to look for signs of illness or injury. Focus the examination around:

+ What the person (or others in the area) have told you.

+ How the person is acting.

+ What you see.

Check the part of the body that the person is saying hurts, is holding, or where you see obvious signs of injury, including bleeding, cuts, burns, bruising, swelling or deformities. The person may have multiple signs of an injury or illness in different areas of their body. In this case, do a focused examination of each of these areas.

To perform a focused examination, look and gently feel for signs of injury. Think of how the body normally looks. If you are unsure if a body part or limb is injured, check it against the opposite limb or other side of the body. Watch the person's face for expressions of discomfort or pain as you feel for injuries. Note if the person cannot feel you touching the body part or if touching the area causes pain. If the person experiences pain, stop checking that area. Check the person's ability to move the body part unless they are unable or unwilling to move it.

> ## ⓘ CARE ALERT!
>
> Do not ask the person to move if you suspect a head, neck or spinal injury.

While you are checking the person, notice how their skin looks and feels. Is their skin pale, gray (ashen), blue (cyanotic) or flushed? Does it feel moist or dry, cool or hot? Also take note of any medical identification tags (typically worn around the neck, wrist or ankle).

2:3 CARE

Provide care consistent with your knowledge and training for the conditions found during the rapid and secondary assessments. Always address life-threatening conditions first. Other professional rescuers and safety team members should assist, either by getting equipment and activating the EMS system (Box 2-4) or in the actual delivery of care (for example, providing two-rescuer CPR and using an AED). Give appropriate care until:

+ Other trained responders or EMS professionals arrive and begin their care of the person.

+ You are too exhausted to continue.

+ The scene becomes unsafe.

In most cases, you should care for the person where they are found. Unnecessary movement can cause additional injury and pain and may complicate the person's recovery. It may be appropriate to move a person under the following three conditions:

+ You must move the person to protect them from immediate danger.

+ You must move the person to reach another person who may have a more serious injury or illness.

+ You must move the person to give proper care. For example, it may be necessary to move a person to a hard, flat surface to provide CPR or control life-threatening bleeding.

Box 2-4 IF YOU ARE ALONE IN AN EMERGENCY

Most of the time when you are working as a professional rescuer, you will be working as part of a team and one team member will summon emergency medical services (EMS) while other team members provide care. But what should you do if you are alone with the person and there is no one to send to call EMS?

If you are **alone** and **you have a mobile phone** available near you, make the call quickly and put the dispatcher on speaker phone so that you can begin care.

If you are **alone** and you **do not have a mobile phone** available, you should summon EMS and then provide care in most cases. Activate the EMS system quickly so that you can return to the person and begin providing care as soon as possible. However, in the following situations, you should give immediate care and then go activate the EMS system.

+ The person has drowned.

+ The person is an unresponsive infant or a child younger than about 12 years and you did not see them collapse.

+ The person is choking.

+ The person is experiencing a severe allergic reaction (anaphylaxis) and has an epinephrine auto-injector.

+ The person has life-threatening bleeding.

In these situations, there are actions that you can take right away that may prevent the person's condition from worsening. After you take these actions, call 9-1-1 or the designated emergency number to get EMS on the way.

If you must move a person, the goal is to do so without injuring yourself or causing additional injury to the person (Box 2-5).

Box 2-5 EMERGENCY MOVES

There are several ways to move a person. Choose a method according to the situation. Always use good body mechanics to avoid injury to yourself. Avoid twisting or bending anyone who has a possible head, neck or spinal injury.

Move	When to Use It	How to Do It
Walking Assist	To move a person who can walk but needs help	1. Place the person's arm around your shoulder or waist and hold it in place with one hand. 2. Support the person with your other hand around their waist.
Two-Person Seat Carry	To move a responsive person who is not seriously injured Do not use if you suspect a head, neck or spinal injury	1. Put one arm under the person's thighs and the other across their back, under their arms. Have a second rescuer do the same. 2. Interlock your arms with the other rescuer's arms under the person's legs and across the person's back. 3. Lift the person in the "seat" formed by your interlocked arms.
Clothes Drag	To move a responsive or unresponsive person who may have a head, neck or back injury	1. Grasp the person's shirt behind the neck, gathering enough material so that you have a firm grip. 2. Cradle the person's head with the shirt and your hands and, keeping their head midline without lifting it, pull them to safety.

2:4 WRAP-UP

When responding to any emergency, your priorities are to ensure your own safety, as well as the safety of others in the area, and to take appropriate action to address life-threatening conditions first. In any emergency, perform a rapid assessment to ensure safety and identify and care for life-threatening conditions. When the person's condition allows, perform a secondary assessment.

 BENCHMARK SUMMARY

Benchmarks for Professional Rescuers

Professional rescuers should:

+ Conduct a rapid assessment for timely determination of life-threatening conditions.

Opening the Airway

Head-Tilt/Chin-Lift Technique

1   Kneel to the side of the person's head.

2   Press down on the forehead while pulling up on the bony part of the chin with two to three fingers of your other hand.

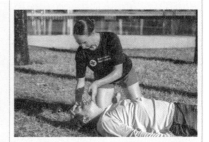

3   Tilt the head back as you lift up on the chin.
- **Adult:** Tilt the head to a past-neutral position.
- **Child:** Tilt the head to a slightly past-neutral position.
- **Infant:** Tilt the head to a neutral position.

Jaw-Thrust Maneuver with Head Extension

1   Kneel above the person's head.

2   Put one hand on either side of the person's head, with your thumbs near the corners of the mouth and pointed toward the chin. Slide your fingers under the angles of the jawbone.

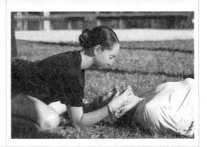

Continued

| 3 | Thrust the jaw up and tilt the head back to open the airway.

 • **Adult:** Tilt the head to a past-neutral position.

 • **Child:** Tilt the head to a slightly past-neutral position.

 • **Infant:** Tilt the head to a neutral position. | |

Modified Jaw-Thrust Maneuver

1	Kneel above the person's head.	
2	Put one hand on either side of the person's head, with your thumbs near the corners of the mouth and pointed toward the chin. Slide your fingers under the angles of the jawbone **without moving the person's head or neck.**	
3	Thrust the jaw up **(again without moving the head or neck)** to lift the jaw and open the airway.	

Skill Sheet 2-2. Rapid Assessment

1 Perform a scene size-up.

- Make sure the environment is safe—for you, your team and anyone else there.

- Gather an initial impression of the person, which includes looking for life-threatening bleeding.

- Quickly determine the need for additional resources.

NOTE! If there is life-threatening bleeding, control it with any available resources (including the use of a tourniquet or hemostatic dressing as appropriate) and, if not already done, make sure EMS has been called.

Continued

2 Check for responsiveness.

- Shout, "Are you OK?" Use the person's name if you know it.

- Tap the person's shoulders (for an **adult or child**) or the bottom of the person's foot (for an **infant**) and shout again (shout-tap-shout).

- If the person is unresponsive, make sure EMS has been called if you have not already done so.

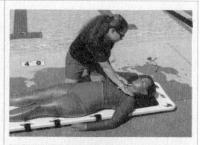

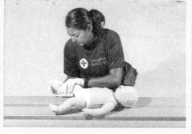

Continued

3 Simultaneously check for breathing, a pulse and life-threatening bleeding.

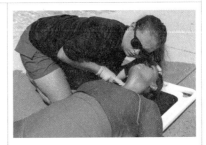

- Make sure the person is in a supine (face-up) position. If they are face-down, roll them onto their back, taking care not to create or worsen a suspected injury.
- To open the airway:

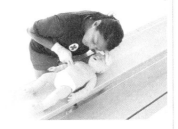

  - From the side, use the head-tilt/chin-lift technique.
  - From above the person's head, use the jaw-thrust with head extension maneuver.
  - If a head, neck or spinal injury is suspected, use the modified jaw-thrust maneuver.
- Simultaneously check for breathing and a pulse for no more than 10 seconds.
  - **Adult or child:** Feel for a carotid pulse by placing two fingers in the middle of the person's throat and sliding them into the groove at the side of the neck closest to you.
  - **Infant:** Feel for a brachial pulse on the inside of the upper arm between the infant's elbow and shoulder.
- At the same time, scan the body for life-threatening bleeding.

Continued

4 Give 2 ventilations to a person who is not breathing as a result of drowning.

- Each ventilation should last about 1 second and make the chest begin to rise; allow the air to exit before delivering the next ventilation.

- If either ventilation is unsuccessful, reopen the airway, make a seal and try another ventilation for a total of 2 initial ventilations.

- Do not attempt more than 3 ventilations before beginning care.

Continued

5 Provide care based on the conditions found.

- If the person is not breathing (or is breathing ineffectively) but has a pulse, give ventilations.
  - **Adult:** Provide 1 ventilation every 6 seconds.
  - **Child and infant:** Provide 1 ventilation every 2 to 3 seconds.
- If the person is not breathing normally (or is only gasping) and has no pulse, begin CPR immediately, starting with compressions, and use an AED as soon as it is available.
- If the person is unresponsive but breathing or responsive but not fully awake, place them in the recovery position.
  - Extend the person's arm that is closest to you above the person's head.
  - Roll the person toward yourself onto their side, so that the person's head rests on their extended arm.
  - Bend both of the person's knees to stabilize their body.

NOTE! If you suspect a head, neck or spinal injury, leave the person in a face-up position unless you are unable to maintain an open airway.

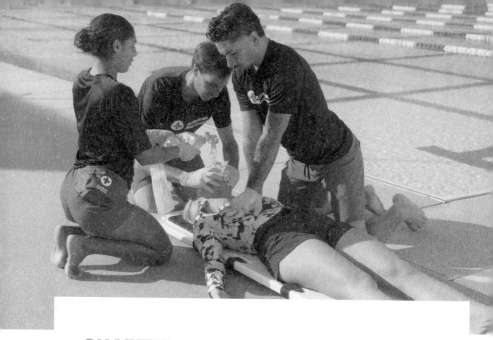

CHAPTER 3
VENTILATIONS AND AIRWAY MANAGEMENT

Because oxygen is essential for life, you must always make sure that
the person has an open airway and is breathing effectively. Breathing,
or ventilation, is the mechanical process of moving air into and out of
the body. If the person is not breathing or is breathing ineffectively,
you will need to provide ventilations after ensuring an open airway. The
airway is the pathway from the mouth and nose to the lungs. If the
airway is not open and clear, oxygen cannot reach the lungs, where it
moves into the bloodstream to be distributed to the rest of the body.
You have already learned how techniques like the head-tilt/chin-lift
technique can be used to open the airway. Depending on the situation,
you may also need to use tools (such as suctioning or a basic airway
device) to maintain an open airway, or techniques to clear the airway
(such as back blows and abdominal thrusts).

3:1 THE RESPIRATORY SYSTEM

The function of the respiratory system is to provide the body's cells with oxygen and to remove the byproduct of cellular metabolism, carbon dioxide. **Respiration** (the process of moving oxygen and carbon dioxide between the atmosphere and the body's cells) includes **ventilation** (the mechanical process of moving air into and out of the body) and **gas exchange** (the molecular process of adding oxygen to, and removing carbon dioxide from, the blood). Effective respiration relies on effective functioning of the respiratory system, the cardiovascular system and the nervous system.

Hypoxia (low oxygen levels in the body's tissues) can occur as a result of conditions that affect the respiratory, cardiovascular or neurologic systems and, if not addressed, can lead to impaired organ function and death. For example, when the brain is deprived of oxygen, brain damage can begin in as little as 4 to 6 minutes. After 8 to 10 minutes with insufficient oxygen, brain damage can become irreversible (Figure 3-1). Many different conditions can lead to hypoxia, including drowning, choking (airway obstruction), cardiac arrest and conditions that cause respiratory compromise.

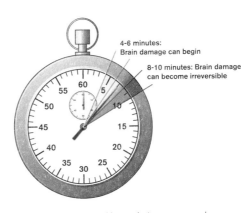

4-6 minutes: Brain damage can begin

8-10 minutes: Brain damage can become irreversible

Figure 3-1. Time is critical in respiratory emergencies.

3:2 RESPIRATORY COMPROMISE

Respiratory compromise (a decrease in respiratory function) is progressive, which means that if the person does not receive care quickly, their respiratory function will become increasingly worse (Figure 3-2).

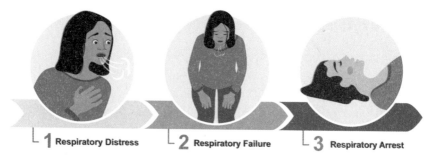

Figure 3-2 Respiratory distress can lead to respiratory failure, which in turn can lead to respiratory arrest. If not addressed, respiratory arrest leads to cardiac arrest.

+ Respiratory distress, or difficulty breathing, is the earliest stage of respiratory compromise. Many conditions can cause respiratory distress, including acute flare-ups of chronic respiratory conditions (such as asthma), severe allergic reactions (anaphylaxis), lung and respiratory tract infections, heart conditions (such as a heart attack or heart failure), trauma, poisoning, drug overdose and mental health conditions (such as panic disorder). The person's work of breathing is increased, but ventilation and gas exchange are still adequate to meet the body's demands.

+ If respiratory distress is not relieved, respiratory failure can occur. In respiratory failure, the respiratory system is beginning to shut down. There may be some ventilation, but it is not sufficient to sustain gas exchange and as a result, the blood contains too little oxygen, too much carbon dioxide, or both.

+ If respiratory failure is not relieved, respiratory arrest can occur. In respiratory arrest, breathing stops. The body can tolerate respiratory arrest for only a very short time before the heart stops functioning as well, leading to cardiac arrest.

3:3 VENTILATIONS

When a person is not breathing or is breathing ineffectively, you need to provide ventilations for them. You will give ventilations:

+ During the rapid assessment for a person who is not breathing as a result of drowning.

+ When caring for a person in respiratory arrest or respiratory failure.

+ When providing CPR to a person in cardiac arrest.

Table 3-1 summarizes information about giving ventilations for each of these conditions.

When giving ventilations, remember these key points:

+ Use a resuscitation mask or bag-valve-mask (BVM) resuscitator.

+ Maintain an open airway using the head-tilt/chin-lift technique, the jaw-thrust maneuver with head extension or the modified jaw-thrust maneuver.

+ Position and seal the mask properly over the person's mouth and nose.

+ Avoid excessive ventilation. Each ventilation should last about 1 second and make the person's chest begin to rise. Allow the chest to fall before delivering the next ventilation.

Using proper technique is important when giving ventilations. If you give too much air or you deliver the air too quickly or with too much force, complications may result. For example, increased airway pressure can cause air to enter the stomach, leading to gastric distension and increasing the risk for vomiting and aspiration.

Box 3-1 describes how to manage special situations when giving ventilations.

Table 3-1 Giving Ventilations

Condition	When to Give Ventilations	Pacing of Ventilations	Notes
Drowning (person not breathing)	Give 2 initial ventilations as part of the rapid assessment.	• Give 1 ventilation, pause briefly to allow person's chest to fall, then give another ventilation.	• If the chest does not rise after either the first or second ventilation, reopen the airway, make a seal, and try another ventilation for a total of 2 initial ventilations. • Do not attempt more than 3 ventilations before beginning care.
Respiratory arrest or respiratory failure	Give ventilations if the person is not breathing (or is breathing ineffectively) but has a pulse. • Give ventilations for about 2 minutes, then check for breathing and a pulse. • If the person is still not breathing but has a pulse, continue giving ventilations for another 2 minutes and then check again for breathing and a pulse. • If at any time the person does not have a pulse, begin CPR immediately.	• **Adults:** 1 ventilation every 6 seconds • **Children and infants:** 1 ventilation every 2 to 3 seconds	• If the chest does not rise after a ventilation, reopen the airway, make a seal, and try another ventilation. If the chest does not rise after the additional attempt, provide care for a potential airway obstruction by immediately beginning CPR, starting with compressions.
Cardiac arrest	Give 2 ventilations after every set of compressions.	• Give 1 ventilation, pause briefly to allow the person's chest to fall, then give another ventilation.	• If the chest does not rise after the first ventilation, reopen the airway, make a seal, and try another ventilation. • Do not attempt more than 2 ventilations before resuming compressions. If the chest does not rise after the additional attempt, provide care for a potential airway obstruction. • The process of giving 2 ventilations and then resuming compressions should take less than 10 seconds.

Box 3-1 MANAGING SPECIFIC SITUATIONS THAT MAY ARISE WHEN GIVING VENTILATIONS

The Person Vomits

When you give ventilations, the person may vomit. Many people who have been submerged vomit because water has entered the stomach or air has been forced accidentally into the stomach during ventilations. If the person starts to vomit while you are giving ventilations, quickly turn them onto their side to prevent the vomit from blocking the airway and entering the lungs. Clear the person's airway using a gloved finger and, if one is available and you are trained to use it, a suctioning device. Then roll the person onto their back and continue giving care.

The Person Has a Suspected Head, Neck or Spinal Injury

If you suspect that a person who is not breathing has a head, neck or spinal injury, always take care of the airway and breathing first. If the person is on a backboard, remove the head immobilizer device and forehead strap before opening the airway. Open the airway using the modified jaw-thrust maneuver. If the modified jaw-thrust maneuver does not open the airway, use the jaw-thrust maneuver with head extension or the head-tilt/chin-lift technique. If the person vomits, tilt the backboard or quickly roll the person onto their side while supporting the head and neck and turning the person's body as a unit. Clear the person's airway, then roll the person onto their back and continue giving care.

The Person Has a Stoma

Some people may breathe through a **stoma** (a surgically created opening in the neck). To give ventilations to a person with a stoma, keep the airway in a neutral position and make an airtight

Continued

Box 3-1 MANAGING SPECIFIC SITUATIONS THAT MAY ARISE WHEN GIVING VENTILATIONS (Continued)

seal with a round infant resuscitation mask around the stoma or tracheostomy tube.

You Do Not Have Equipment

If you do not have a resuscitation mask or a bag-valve-mask (BVM) resuscitator, provide mouth-to-mouth ventilations.

Use the head-tilt/chin-lift technique to open the airway. With the person's head tilted back, pinch the nose shut. Take a normal breath, make a complete seal over the person's mouth with your mouth and blow into the person's mouth to deliver 1 ventilation over 1 second until you see the chest begin to rise. After each ventilation, break the seal and take a breath before resealing your mouth over the person's mouth. Then deliver the next ventilation.

The oxygen concentration of ambient air is approximately 20%. With mouth-to-mouth ventilations, the air the person receives contains approximately 16% to 17% oxygen. Breaking the seal after each ventilation and taking a breath can help maintain an oxygen concentration of approximately 16% to 17%. If you do not break the seal and take a breath between ventilations, the second ventilation may contain a lower oxygen concentration and a high concentration of carbon dioxide.

You Are Unable to Form a Tight Seal Over the Person's Mouth

Use mouth-to-nose ventilations if you are unable to form a tight seal over the person's mouth (for example, due to an injury). Use the head-tilt/chin-lift technique to open the airway. With the person's head tilted back, close the mouth by pushing up on the chin. Seal your mouth around the person's nose and breathe into the nose. If possible, open the person's mouth between ventilations to allow air to escape.

Using a Resuscitation Mask

Resuscitation masks have a one-way valve that prevents the rescuer from inhaling air exhaled by the person, and they may also have an oxygen inlet that can be connected to an emergency oxygen source (Figure 3-3). The style of the mask may vary slightly.

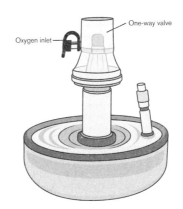

Figure 3-3 A resuscitation mask has a one-way valve that prevents the rescuer from breathing air exhaled by the person. Some resuscitation masks also have an inlet for delivering emergency oxygen.

+ In aquatic settings, round "blob"-style resuscitation masks (Figure 3-4A) are common. These masks are easy to place and use in and around water or on land. This style of mask is one-size-fits-all for adults and children older than 18 months.

+ Other styles of resuscitation masks are more pear-shaped (Figure 3-4B). This style of resuscitation mask has a one-way valve with a filter that should be replaced if it gets wet. These masks are sized specifically for adults, children and infants and you must use a mask that is sized appropriately for the person to ensure a proper fit and tight seal.

Whatever style of resuscitation mask you are using, always follow the manufacturer's recommendations for use. Skill Sheet 3-1 describes how to give ventilations using a resuscitation mask.

A   B

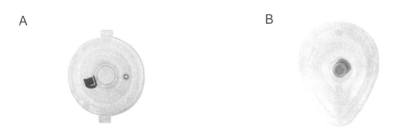

Figure 3-4 (A) A round resuscitation mask. (B) A pear-shaped resuscitation mask.

Using a Bag-Valve-Mask Resuscitator

A BVM resuscitator is a hand-held device used to give ventilations. The BVM resuscitator has a mask that is connected by a one-way valve to a self-inflating chamber, or "bag." Squeezing the bag with the mask properly sealed over the person's mouth and nose forces air into the person's lungs. Releasing the bag causes it to self-inflate by drawing air in from the other end. A BVM

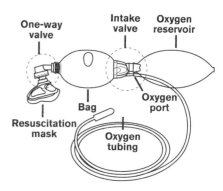

Figure 3-5 A BVM resuscitator has a bag, a one-way valve and a mask and can be connected to emergency oxygen.

resuscitator can be used with or without emergency oxygen. There is an oxygen inlet for attaching the resuscitator to an emergency oxygen source and a reservoir that fills with oxygen (Figure 3-5).

BVM resuscitators are sized specifically for adults, children and infants (Figure 3-6). Always use a BVM resuscitator that is sized appropriately for the person. Using an adult-sized BVM on an infant has the potential to cause harm.

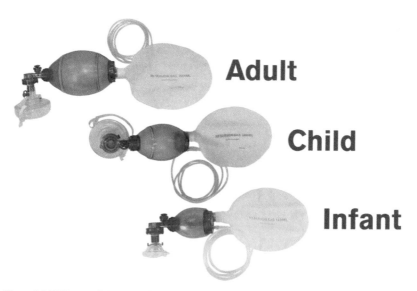

Figure 3-6 BVM resuscitators come in a variety of sizes for use with adults, children and infants.

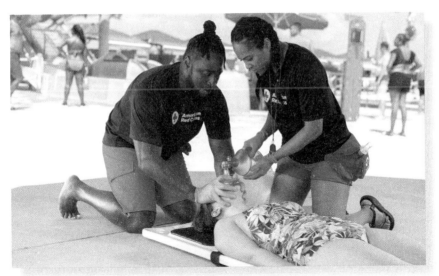

Figure 3-7 Two rescuers are needed to most effectively operate a BVM resuscitator. One rescuer seals the mask and opens the airway, while the other rescuer squeezes the bag to deliver ventilations.

Two rescuers are needed to most effectively operate a BVM resuscitator. One rescuer seals the mask and opens the airway, while the other rescuer squeezes the bag to deliver ventilations (Figure 3-7). To minimize complications when using a BVM resuscitator, depress the bag slowly (over 1 second) and only about halfway to deliver the minimal amount of air. Skill Sheet 3-2 describes how to give ventilations using a BVM resuscitator.

3:4 AIRWAY MANAGEMENT

The airway is the pathway for air to pass between the mouth and nose and the lungs. Without an open and clear airway, oxygen cannot reach the lungs for distribution to the rest of the body. The airway can become blocked by fluids (such as saliva or mucus), foreign matter (such as vomit) or the person's tongue. You have already learned simple measures for keeping the airway open and clear, such as positioning (for example, placing an unresponsive person who is breathing in the recovery position) and manual maneuvers (for example, the head-tilt/chin-lift technique and the jaw-thrust maneuver). Depending on state and local laws and your facility's protocols, you may also be trained in additional techniques for clearing the airway and maintaining an open airway, such as suctioning or the use of a basic airway device.

Suctioning

Suctioning is used to clear the upper airway of excessive secretions, vomit or blood (Figure 3-8).

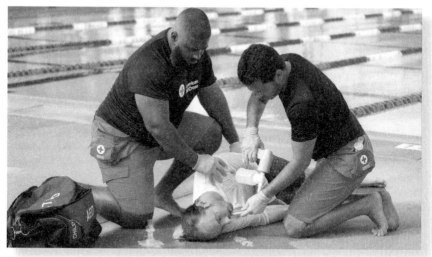

Figure 3-8 Suctioning devices are used to clear a person's upper airway.

> ## ⓘ CARE ALERT
>
> If you observe frothing in a person who has drowned, do not delay care by taking time to suction it. The froth is not blocking the airway and does not need to be suctioned.

> ## ⓘ CARE ALERT
>
> Suctioning should *not* be used in an attempt to remove water from the lungs of a person who has drowned.

Suctioning is performed using a catheter that is attached via tubing to a suction unit, which may be manually operated or electrically powered. Squeezing the handle of a manual suction unit or powering on a mechanical suction unit creates a suction force that is used to remove secretions and foreign matter from the airway.

Manual suction units are lightweight, compact and relatively inexpensive. Because they do not require an energy source, they avoid some of the problems associated with electrically powered units and are well suited for use in an aquatic environment. Mechanical units must be plugged into an electrical outlet, or they may operate on batteries that should be kept fully charged. Both types of suctioning devices use suction catheters, which must be sized appropriately for the person. If suctioning is part of your facility's protocols, there should be several sizes of suction catheters on hand.

Skill Sheet 3-3 describes how to use a suctioning device.

Basic Airways

Basic airways are devices that are inserted through the person's mouth or nose to keep the airway clear and provide a channel for air movement and suctioning. Basic airways must be sized appropriately for the person. Once the basic airway is in place, you can use a resuscitation mask or a BVM resuscitator to provide ventilations as you normally would. When providing ventilations to a person with a basic airway in place, you must still maintain an open airway using the head-tilt/chin-lift technique or the jaw-thrust maneuver.

Oropharyngeal Airway

An **oropharyngeal airway (OPA)** is inserted through the person's mouth. The curved body of the airway fits over the tongue and holds it up and away from the back of the throat (Figure 3-9A). An OPA should only be used in an unresponsive person. Do not use an OPA in a responsive person with intact cough or gag reflexes. In addition, avoid using an OPA in a person with oral trauma.

Nasopharyngeal Airway

A **nasopharyngeal airway (NPA)** is a soft rubber tube with a flange on one end and a beveled tip on the other. The NPA is inserted through the nose and extends to the back of the throat to provide a channel for air movement and suctioning (Figure 3-9B). An NPA may be used in a responsive or unresponsive person. Do not use an NPA in a person with

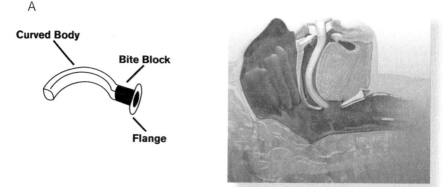

A

Curved Body

Bite Block

Flange

B

Flange

Beveled
Tip

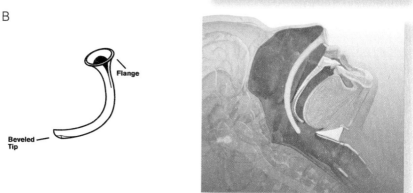

Figure 3-9 Basic airways are inserted through the person's mouth or nose to keep the airway clear and provide a channel for air movement and suctioning. (**A**) An oropharyngeal airway. (**B**) A nasopharyngeal airway.

a possible skull or facial fracture. Exercise caution if considering use of an NPA in a person with suspected head trauma.

3:5 EMERGENCY OXYGEN

The percentage of oxygen in the air a person normally breathes is about 21%. When giving ventilations with a resuscitation mask, the air exhaled by the rescuer (and inhaled by the person) contains about 16% oxygen. When giving ventilations with a BVM resuscitator, the air the person receives contains the normal concentration of oxygen, about 21%. Emergency oxygen increases the oxygen content of the air provided to the person.

Emergency oxygen can be administered to responsive or unresponsive people, as well as to people who are breathing on their own and those who are receiving ventilations (for example, with a BVM resuscitator). Administering emergency oxygen to a person experiencing a breathing emergency can help improve hypoxia (Figure 3-10). It can also reduce pain and breathing discomfort. Emergency oxygen can be given for many breathing and cardiac emergencies but should only be administered as a secondary treatment after the priorities of airway management, ventilation, CPR, use of an AED and bleeding control have been addressed. Always follow local protocols for using emergency oxygen.

Skill Sheet 3-4 describes how to administer emergency oxygen. When preparing and administering oxygen, safety is a priority (Box 3-2).

Oxygen Delivery Systems

Oxygen delivery systems may be variable-flow-rate systems or fixed-flow-rate systems.

Variable-Flow-Rate Systems

Variable-flow-rate systems allow the rescuer to adjust the flow of oxygen based on the person's need. The flow can generally be set from 1 to 15 liters per minute (LPM). Variable-flow-rate oxygen systems must be assembled by the rescuer and include an oxygen cylinder, a pressure regulator with a pressure gauge and flowmeter, and an oxygen delivery device.

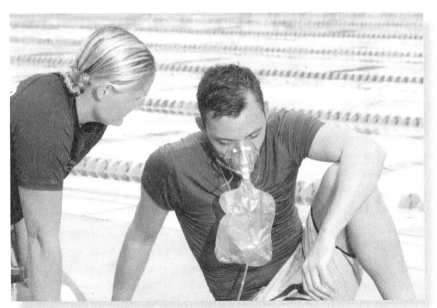

Figure 3-10 Emergency oxygen increases the oxygen content of the air the person breathes and can help improve or eliminate hypoxia.

Box 3-2 OXYGEN SAFETY PRECAUTIONS

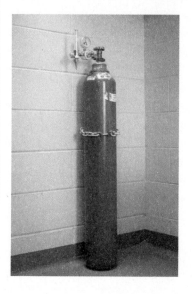

Always use oxygen equipment according to the manufacturer's instructions and in a manner consistent with federal and local regulations.

+ Oxygen cylinders are under high pressure and must be handled carefully. Do not carry a cylinder by the valve or pressure regulator. Do not hold on to the protective valve caps or guards when moving or lifting cylinders. Do not drag or roll cylinders. Do not drop cylinders. Do not stand oxygen cylinders upright unless they are well secured. If the cylinder falls, the pressure regulator or valve could become damaged or cause injury due to the intense pressure in the tank.

+ Check for cylinder leaks, abnormal bulging, and defective or inoperative valves or safety devices. Check for rust or corrosion on the cylinder or cylinder neck. Check for foreign substances and residues (such as adhesive tape residue) around the cylinder neck, oxygen valve or regulator assembly. The presence of defects and foreign substances can hamper oxygen delivery, cause a fire or explosion, or both.

+ Be aware of the specific testing requirements for steel and aluminum cylinders (for example, 10 years after initial testing for steel cylinders and 5 years for aluminum cylinders).

+ Ensure that all oxygen cylinders have undergone hydrostatic testing (to verify that they can hold the maximum fill pressure) within the prescribed time frame and that they are marked appropriately.

Continued

Box 3-2 OXYGEN SAFETY PRECAUTIONS (Continued)

+ Do not use oxygen around flames or sparks, including smoking materials such as cigarettes, cigars and pipes. Oxygen causes fire to burn more rapidly and intensely.

+ Do not use grease, oil or petroleum products to lubricate or clean the pressure regulator. This could cause an explosion.

+ Do not deface, alter or remove any labeling or markings on the oxygen cylinder.

+ Do not attempt to mix gases in an oxygen cylinder or transfer oxygen from one cylinder to another. When the oxygen cylinder is empty, close the cylinder valve, replace the valve protection cap or outlet plug (if provided), mark or tag the cylinder as empty, and promptly return the cylinder to be refilled according to state, local and facility regulations and policies.

+ Do not use an AED or manual defibrillator around flammable materials, such as free-flowing oxygen or gasoline. If oxygen is being administered to a person when an AED is ready to be used, make sure the cylinder valve is closed before shocking.

Oxygen cylinder

Medical-grade oxygen cylinders come in various sizes and pressure capacities. They are labeled "U.S.P." and marked with a yellow diamond containing the word "Oxygen" (Figure 3-11). In the United States, oxygen cylinders typically have green markings, but the color scheme is not regulated so different manufacturers and different countries may use different color markings.

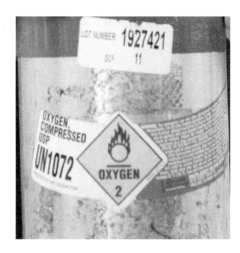

Figure 3-11 Oxygen cylinders are marked with a yellow diamond that reads "Oxygen" and, in the United States, typically have green markings.

Pressure regulator and flowmeter

The pressure regulator reduces the pressure of the oxygen to a safe level. The pressure regulator has a pressure gauge that shows the pressure in the cylinder and allows you to determine how full the cylinder is (Figure 3-12). A full cylinder will show 2000 pounds per square inch (psi), while a nearly empty cylinder will show about 200 psi. A pressure regulator typically has two metal prongs that fit into the valve at the top of the oxygen cylinder (Figure 3-13). An O-ring gasket ensures a tight seal between the pressure regulator and the oxygen cylinder.

The flowmeter controls how rapidly the oxygen flows from the cylinder to the person.

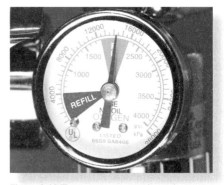

Figure 3-12 The pressure gauge shows the pressure in the cylinder and allows you to determine how full the cylinder is.

Oxygen delivery device

The oxygen delivery device is the piece of equipment the person breathes through when receiving oxygen. Tubing carries the oxygen from the pressure regulator to the delivery device. When delivering oxygen,

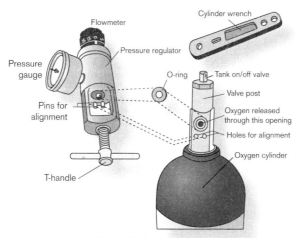

Figure 3-13 The pressure regulator is attached to the oxygen cylinder.

make sure the tubing does not get tangled or kinked because this will slow or stop the flow of oxygen to the delivery device.

The maximum flow rate and concentration of oxygen that can be delivered vary according to the delivery device (Table 3-2). Factors that influence the choice of delivery device include whether the person is spontaneously breathing or requires assisted ventilation with a BVM resuscitator, the desired oxygen concentration, equipment availability and the person's comfort.

Oxygen delivery devices come in sizes appropriate for adults, children and infants. Use an oxygen delivery device that is sized appropriately for the person. Always make sure the oxygen is flowing before putting the delivery device over the person's face.

Nasal cannula. A nasal cannula is only suitable for use on a spontaneously breathing person. The nasal cannula is held in place over the person's ears and oxygen is delivered through two small prongs inserted into the nostrils.

The nasal cannula is commonly used for people with only minor breathing difficulty or for those who have a history of respiratory disease. It is also useful for people who cannot tolerate a face mask. Nasal cannulas are not typically used for people experiencing a serious breathing emergency because these people generally breathe through the mouth and need a device that can supply a greater concentration of oxygen.

Table 3-2 Oxygen Delivery Devices

Delivery Device	Description	Oxygen Flow Rate (LPM)	Oxygen Concentration (%)	Use for a Person Who Is:
Nasal cannula	Held in place over the person's ears; oxygen is delivered through two small prongs inserted into the nostrils	1–6	24–44	Breathing
Simple oxygen face mask	Pliable, dome-shaped mask that fits over the mouth and nose with an oxygen inlet and side ports to permit egress of exhaled gas	6–15	35–55	Breathing
Nonrebreather mask	Face mask with an attached oxygen reservoir bag and one-way valve between the mask and bag; person inhales oxygen from the bag, and exhaled air escapes through flutter valves on the side of the mask	10–15	Up to 90	Breathing
BVM resuscitator	Handheld breathing device consisting of a self-inflating bag, a one-way valve, a face mask and an oxygen reservoir bag	≥ 15	≥ 90	Breathing or not breathing

Simple oxygen face mask. Simple oxygen face masks can deliver high-flow oxygen. However, because room air is drawn in through the side ports and, potentially, around the mask, delivered oxygen concentrations are in the range of 35% to 55%.

Some simple oxygen masks have elastic straps that are placed over the person's head to keep the mask in place. If the mask does not have straps, you or the person can hold the mask in place. A young child or infant may be frightened by having a mask placed on their face. If this is the case, you can use the "blow-by" technique. To use the blow-by technique, hold (or have the child's parent or guardian hold) the mask about 2 inches away from the child's face and wave it slowly from side to side, allowing the oxygen to pass over the face and be inhaled.

Nonrebreather mask. A nonrebreather mask is used to deliver high concentrations of oxygen to a person who is breathing on their own. The one-way valve prevents exhaled air from mixing with the oxygen in the reservoir bag. The person inhales oxygen from the bag and exhaled air escapes through flutter valves on the side of the mask. To inflate the reservoir bag, block the one-way valve with your gloved thumb before placing the mask on the person's face. The oxygen reservoir bag should be sufficiently inflated (about two-thirds full) so it does not deflate when the person inhales. If the bag deflates, increase the flow rate of the oxygen to refill the reservoir bag.

Bag-valve-mask resuscitator. A BVM resuscitator can be used on a breathing or nonbreathing person. A BVM resuscitator with an oxygen reservoir bag is capable of supplying an oxygen concentration of 90% or more when used at a flow rate of 15 LPM or more. As when using a nonrebreather mask, block the one-way valve before applying the mask to allow the reservoir to fill with oxygen.

Fixed-Flow-Rate Systems

Fixed-flow-rate systems have a flow rate that cannot be adjusted. Most fixed-flow-rate tanks are set at 15 LPM; however, you may see tanks set at 6 LPM, 12 LPM or another rate. Some fixed-flow-rate systems have a dual (high/low) flow setting.

Fixed-flow-rate systems typically come with the delivery device, regulator and cylinder already assembled (Figure 3-14), which makes it quick and simple to administer emergency oxygen. To operate a fixed-flow-rate system, simply turn it on according to the manufacturer's instructions, check that the oxygen is flowing and place the delivery device on the person.

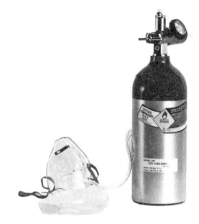

Figure 3-14 Fixed-flow-rate oxygen delivery systems usually come already assembled.

Because the flow rate cannot be adjusted in a fixed-flow-rate system, the concentration of oxygen that can be delivered is limited. These systems can only be used with certain delivery devices as well. For example, a fixed-flow-rate unit with a preset flow rate of 6 LPM can be used only with a nasal cannula or a simple oxygen face mask, whereas a system with a preset flow rate of 12 LPM can be used only with a simple oxygen face mask or a nonrebreather mask.

Monitoring Oxygen Therapy

Pulse oximetry is used to measure how much oxygen the blood is carrying, referred to as the oxygen saturation, and to monitor oxygen therapy. A normal oxygen saturation is approximately 95% to 99%. A reading below 94% may indicate hypoxia (Table 3-3).

Table 3-3 Pulse Oximetry for Guiding Oxygen Therapy

	Pulse Oximetry Reading (Oxygen Saturation)	Oxygen Delivery Device
Normal	95%–100%	N/A
Mild hypoxia	91%–94%	Nasal cannula or simple oxygen face mask
Moderate hypoxia	86%–90%	Nonrebreather mask or bag-valve-mask (BVM) resuscitator
Severe hypoxia	≤ 85%	Nonrebreather mask or bag-valve-mask (BVM) resuscitator

To use a pulse oximeter, position an appropriately sized probe on a finger, toe or earlobe according to the manufacturer's instructions (Figure 3-15). Let the machine register the oxygen saturation level. Verify the person's pulse rate on the oximeter with the person's actual pulse. Oxygen therapy is typically adjusted to achieve an oxygen saturation of at least 94% on pulse oximetry. When monitoring a responsive person's oxygen saturation levels using a pulse oximeter, you may decrease the flow rate of oxygen and change

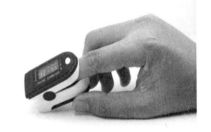

Figure 3-15 A pulse oximeter can be used to measure how much oxygen the blood is carrying.

to a lower flowing delivery device if the oxygen saturation reaches at least 94%.

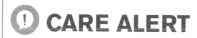

CARE ALERT

Pulse oximetry is an additional assessment tool. The pulse oximetry reading should always be considered in the context of the person's signs and symptoms. It is possible for a person who is having trouble breathing to have a normal pulse oximetry reading. Never withhold oxygen therapy if the person is showing signs and symptoms of respiratory distress or when it is the standard of care to apply oxygen despite good pulse oximetry readings (for example, for a person with chest pain).

3:6 OBSTRUCTED AIRWAY (CHOKING)

An obstructed airway (choking) occurs when the airway becomes either partially or completely blocked by a foreign object (for example, a piece of food, a small toy, or body fluids, such as vomit or blood). Airway obstructions are a common emergency. You need to assess the situation and recognize that a person who cannot speak, cry or cough requires immediate care. If the person does not receive quick and effective care, the airway obstruction can lead to respiratory arrest, which in turn can lead to cardiac arrest.

Recognizing Choking

A responsive person who is choking typically has a panicked, confused or surprised facial expression. Some people may place one or both hands on their throat (Figure 3-16). The person may cough (either forcefully or weakly), or they may not be able to cough at all. You may hear high-pitched squeaking noises as the person tries to breathe, or nothing at all. If the person is making only high-pitched noises or is unable to speak, cry or cough forcefully, the airway is blocked and the person will soon become unresponsive unless the airway is cleared. The person's skin may initially appear flushed (red) but will become pale or bluish in color as the body is deprived of oxygen.

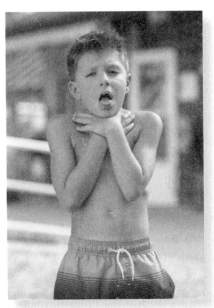

A person who can speak, cry or cough forcefully is getting enough air and the body is trying to clear the obstruction. Encourage an adult or child who is coughing forcefully to continue coughing until they are able to breathe normally and be prepared to intervene if their condition changes. If the person cannot speak or cry or has a weak, ineffective cough, instruct someone to call emergency medical services (EMS) and get equipment and then immediately give care for an obstructed airway.

Figure 3-16 Clutching the throat with one or both hands is commonly referred to as the universal sign of choking.

 CARE ALERT

Remember to obtain consent from the person, or from a child's or infant's parent or guardian. If the parent or guardian is not available, consent is implied.

Obstructed Airway Care (Adult or Child)

Skill Sheet 3-5 describes obstructed airway care for an adult or child.

Responsive Adult or Child

When a responsive adult or child is choking, give a combination of 5 **back blows** (blows between the shoulder blades) followed by 5 **abdominal thrusts** (inward and upward thrusts just above the navel). In some situations, it may be appropriate to give **chest thrusts** instead of abdominal thrusts (Figure 3-17). The goal of giving back blows and

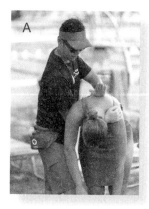 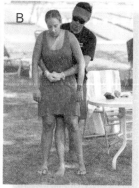 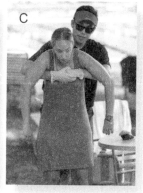

Figure 3-17 Use a combination of (**A**) back blows and (**B**) abdominal thrusts when a responsive adult or child is choking. (**C**) Give chest thrusts instead of abdominal thrusts if back blows and abdominal thrusts are not effective or if you cannot reach around the person to give abdominal thrusts, the person is pregnant or the person is in a wheelchair with features that make it difficult to give abdominal thrusts.

abdominal thrusts (or chest thrusts) is to force the object out of the airway, allowing the person to breathe. Back blows, abdominal thrusts and chest thrusts are all equally effective, but it may take more than one technique to clear the airway.

Give sets of 5 back blows and 5 abdominal thrusts (or chest thrusts) until the person can cough, speak or cry, or until the person becomes unresponsive.

 CARE ALERT

After the choking incident is over, even if the person seems fine, they should be evaluated by a healthcare provider to make sure there is no damage to the airway and to make sure there are no other internal injuries.

Back blows

To give back blows, position yourself to the side and slightly behind the person. For a small child, you may need to kneel. Place one arm diagonally across the person's chest (to provide support) and bend the person forward at the waist so that their upper body is as parallel to the ground as possible. In addition to helping to remove the object, this position allows you to brace yourself if the person becomes unresponsive. Firmly strike the person between the shoulder blades with the heel of your other hand (see Figure 3-17A). Each of the 5 back blows should be separate from the others.

Abdominal thrusts

After the fifth back blow, if the person is unable to cough, speak or cry, give abdominal thrusts. To give abdominal thrusts, have the person stand up straight. Find the person's navel with two fingers, then move behind the person and place your front foot in between the person's feet. Bend your knees slightly to provide balance and stability. For a small child or a person in a wheelchair, you may need to kneel behind them.

Make a fist with your other hand and place the thumb side against the person's abdomen, right above your fingers. Take your first hand and cover your fist with that hand (see Figure 3-17B). Pull inward and upward to give an abdominal thrust. Each of the 5 abdominal thrusts should be separate from the others.

Chest thrusts

For an adult or child, use chest thrusts instead of abdominal thrusts in the following situations:

+ You cannot reach far enough around the person to perform abdominal thrusts.

+ The person is obviously pregnant or known to be pregnant.

+ The person is in a wheelchair with features that make abdominal thrusts difficult to do.

+ Back blows and abdominal thrusts are not effective in dislodging the object.

To give chest thrusts to an adult or child, position yourself behind the person as you would for abdominal thrusts. Make a fist with one hand, place the thumb side of your fist on the center of the person's chest, and cover your fist with the other hand (see Figure 3-17C). Pull inward to give a chest thrust. Each of the 5 chest thrusts should be separate from the others.

Unresponsive Adult or Child

If an adult or child who is choking becomes unresponsive, carefully lower them to a firm, flat surface. Make sure someone has been sent to call EMS and get equipment, if you have not already done so. Immediately begin CPR, starting with chest compressions. (You will learn how to provide CPR to an adult or child in Chapter 4.) Compressions may help clear the airway by moving the blockage into the upper airway, where it can be seen and removed.

After each set of chest compressions and before attempting ventilations, open the person's mouth and look for the object (Figure 3-18A). If you see the object in the person's mouth, remove it using a finger sweep (Figure 3-18B). Next, attempt 2 ventilations. Never try more than 2 ventilations during one cycle of CPR, even if the chest does not rise.

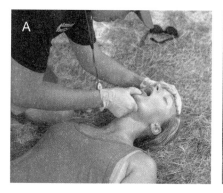 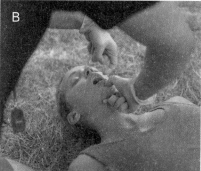

Figure 3-18 If the person becomes unresponsive, (**A**) look for the object in the person's mouth and, if you see it, (**B**) use a finger sweep to remove it.

 CARE ALERT

Only do a finger sweep if you can see the object in the person's mouth. Otherwise, you could accidentally push the object deeper into the person's throat.

If the ventilations go in, resume the normal CPR sequence of compressions and ventilations and use of an AED. If the ventilations do not go in, continue the normal CPR sequence, but check for an object (and remove it if seen) before each set of ventilations.

Obstructed Airway Care (Infant)

Skill Sheet 3-6 describes obstructed airway care for an infant.

Responsive Infant

When a responsive infant is choking, give a combination of 5 back blows followed by 5 chest thrusts (Figure 3-19). You can sit, kneel or stand to give care, as long as you are able to support the infant along your forearm with your arm braced on your thigh and the infant's head lower than their chest. If the infant is large or your hands are small, it may be easier to sit or kneel.

Give sets of 5 back blows and 5 chest thrusts until the infant can cough or cry, or until the infant becomes unresponsive.

Back blows

Place the infant's back along your forearm, cradling the back of the infant's head with your hand. Place your other forearm on the infant's front, supporting the infant's jaw with your thumb and fingers. Be careful not to cover the infant's mouth with your hand while you are supporting the infant's jaw. Turn the infant to a face-down position and hold them along your forearm, using your thigh for support and keeping the infant's

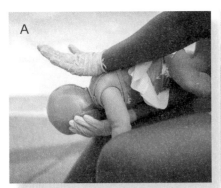
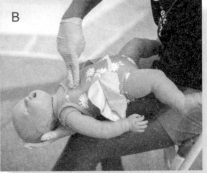

Figure 3-19 Use a combination of (**A**) back blows and (**B**) chest thrusts when a responsive infant is choking.

head lower than their body. Continue to support the infant's jaw with the thumb and fingers of one hand, making sure your fingers are on the sides of the head and not blocking the infant's mouth. Firmly strike the infant between the shoulder blades with the heel of your other hand (see Figure 3-19A). Keep your fingers up to avoid hitting the infant's head or neck. Each of the 5 back blows should be separate from the others.

Chest thrusts

After the fifth back blow, if the infant is unable to cough or cry, give chest thrusts (see Figure 3-19B). Position the infant between your forearms, supporting the head and neck, and turn the infant face-up. Lower the infant onto your thigh with their head lower than their chest. Place two fingers in the center of the infant's chest, just below the nipple line. Give 5 quick chest thrusts about 1½ inches deep. Keep your fingers in contact with the chest, but let the chest return to its normal position after each chest thrust. Each chest thrust should be separate from the others. Remember to support the infant's head, neck and back while giving chest thrusts.

Unresponsive Infant

If an infant who is choking becomes unresponsive, carefully lower them to a firm, flat surface. Make sure someone has been sent to call EMS and get equipment, if you have not already done so. Immediately begin CPR, starting with chest compressions. Use the encircling thumbs technique or the two-finger technique to give chest compressions. (You will learn how to provide CPR to an infant in Chapter 4.)

After each set of chest compressions and before attempting ventilations, open the infant's mouth and look for the object (Figure 3-20A). If you see the object in the infant's mouth, remove it using a finger sweep with your pinky finger (Figure 3-20B). Only do a finger sweep if you can see the object in the infant's mouth. Otherwise, you could accidentally push the object deeper into the infant's throat. Next, attempt 2 ventilations. Never try more than 2 ventilations during one cycle of CPR, even if the chest does not rise.

If the ventilations go in, resume the normal CPR sequence of compressions and ventilations and use of an AED. If the ventilations do not go in, continue the normal CPR sequence, but check for an object (and remove it if seen) before each set of ventilations.

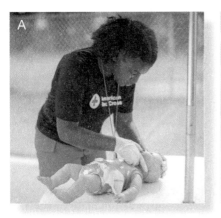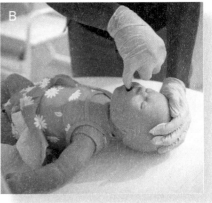

Figure 3-20 If the infant becomes unresponsive, (**A**) look for the object in the infant's mouth and, if you see it, (**B**) remove it with a finger sweep using your pinky finger.

3:7 WRAP-UP

Conditions that impair breathing, including drowning and choking, are life-threatening. Damage to vital organs such as the heart and brain can occur in as little as 4 to 6 minutes when the tissues are deprived of an adequate oxygen supply. Supporting breathing (for example, by giving ventilations) and maintaining a clear airway can be lifesaving.

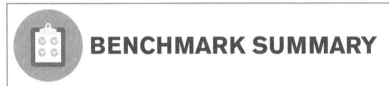

BENCHMARK SUMMARY

Benchmarks for Professional Rescuers

Professional rescuers should:

+ Provide appropriate care for people experiencing respiratory emergencies, which includes:

  – Recognizing that drowning is a respiratory emergency and providing appropriate care.

  – Recognizing and providing care for responsive and unresponsive people with obstructed airways.

  – Handling life-threatening situations with a sense of urgency.

  – Using resuscitation equipment properly, including appropriately sized resuscitation masks and bag-valve-mask (BVM) resuscitators.

  – Administering emergency oxygen using a variety of oxygen delivery devices, if the rescuer is trained and certified in administering emergency oxygen and oxygen delivery is permitted by local protocols.

Giving Ventilations Using a Resuscitation Mask

NOTE! Round resuscitation masks are one-size-fits-all for adults and children older than 18 months. Pear-shaped resuscitation masks are sized specifically for adults, children and infants. Use a mask that is sized appropriately for the person to ensure a proper fit and tight seal.

Head-Tilt/Chin-Lift Technique

1	Kneel to the side of the person's head.	
2	Place the mask. • **Round mask:** Place the mask so that it covers the person's mouth and nose, with the opening over the person's mouth. • **Pear-shaped mask:** Place the mask at the bridge of the nose and lower it over the person's nose and mouth.	

Continued

Giving Ventilations Using a Resuscitation Mask (Continued)

3	Seal the mask and open the airway.
	
	• Place the space between your thumb and index finger at the top of the mask above the one-way valve. Rest your remaining fingers on the side of the person's face.
	
	• Place the thumb of your other hand along the base of the mask and place your bent index finger under the person's chin.
	
	• Lift the person's face into the mask and open the airway by tilting the head back.
	   • **Adult:** past-neutral position
	   • **Child:** slightly past-neutral position
	   • **Infant:** neutral position
		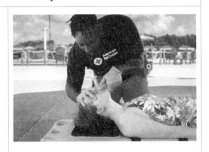

4	Provide ventilations. • Take a normal breath and make a complete seal over the one-way valve. • Blow into the person's mouth for about 1 second, looking to see that the chest begins to rise. • Pause between ventilations to allow the person's chest to fall.	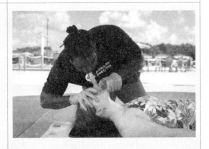

Continued

Giving Ventilations Using a Resuscitation Mask (Continued)

Jaw-Thrust Maneuver with Head Extension

1	Kneel above the person's head.	
2	Place the mask. • **Round mask:** Place the mask so that it covers the person's mouth and nose, with the opening over the person's mouth. • **Pear-shaped mask:** Place the mask at the bridge of the nose and lower it over the person's nose and mouth.	

Continued

Skill Sheet 3-1. Giving Ventilations Using a Resuscitation Mask (Continued)

3	Seal the mask and open the airway.

- **Method A:** Place both hands around the one-way valve, forming a C with your thumb and index finger around the sides of the mask and an E with the last three fingers of each hand under the person's jawbone.

- **Method B:** Place both thumbs along the sides of the one-way valve and your fingers under the person's jawbone.

- Lift the person's face into the mask and open the airway by tilting the head back.
  - **Adult:** past-neutral position
  - **Child:** slightly past-neutral position
  - **Infant:** neutral position

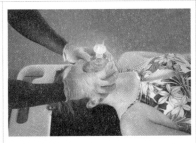

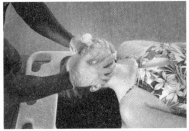

Continued

4	Provide ventilations.	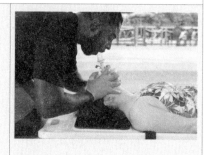
	• Take a normal breath and make a complete seal over the one-way valve.	
	• Blow into the person's mouth for about 1 second, looking to see that the chest begins to rise.	
	• Pause between ventilations to allow the person's chest to fall.	

Continued

Giving Ventilations Using a Resuscitation Mask (Continued)

Modified Jaw-Thrust Maneuver

1	Kneel above the person's head.	
2	Place the mask. • **Round mask:** Place the mask so that it covers the person's mouth and nose, with the opening over the person's mouth. • **Pear-shaped mask:** Place the mask at the bridge of the nose and lower it over the person's nose and mouth.	
3	Seal the mask and open the airway. • **Method A:** Place both hands around the one-way valve, forming a C with your thumb and index finger around the sides of the mask and an E with the last three fingers of each hand under the person's jawbone. • **Method B:** Place both thumbs along the sides of the one-way valve and your fingers under the person's jawbone. • Lift the jaw up **without tilting the head back**.	

Continued

Giving Ventilations Using a Resuscitation Mask (Continued)

4	Provide ventilations.	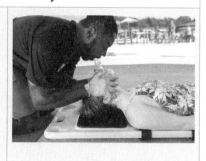

Provide ventilations.

- Take a normal breath and make a complete seal over the one-way valve.

- Blow into the person's mouth for about 1 second, looking to see that the chest begins to rise.

- Pause between ventilations to allow the person's chest to fall.

Giving Ventilations Using a Bag-Valve-Mask Resuscitator

NOTE! Bag-valve-mask (BVM) resuscitators are sized specifically for adults, children and infants. Use a BVM resuscitator that is sized appropriately for the person.

1	Select an appropriately sized BVM resuscitator and assemble it if necessary. • First attach the HEPA filter (if you are using one) to an appropriately sized resuscitation mask. • Attach the bag to the mask assembly.	
2	Place the mask. • The rescuer managing the airway gets into position behind the person's head and places the mask.	

3	The rescuer managing the airway seals the mask and opens the airway.
	     • **Adult:** past-neutral position
	     • **Child:** slightly past-neutral position
	     • **Infant:** neutral position
	
	 NOTE! Use the modified jaw-thrust maneuver if a head, neck or spinal injury is suspected.	

Continued

Skill Sheet 3-2. **Giving Ventilations Using a Bag-Valve-Mask Resuscitator (Continued)**

4	Provide ventilations.	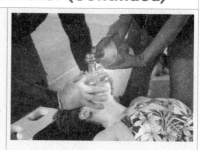
	• The rescuer managing the airway maintains the mask seal and an open airway.	
	• The rescuer giving ventilations gently squeezes the bag about halfway.	
	• The rescuer giving ventilations provides smooth and effortless ventilations that last about 1 second and cause the chest to begin to rise.	
	• Both rescuers watch for chest rise.	

Skill Sheet 3-3. **Using a Suctioning Device**

1	Assemble the device if necessary.	
2	Position the person. • Roll the person's body as a unit onto one side. **NOTE!** If the person has an obvious sign of injury, suction them in the position found, as appropriate.	
3	Open the person's mouth and remove any visible large debris from the mouth with a gloved finger if the person is unresponsive.	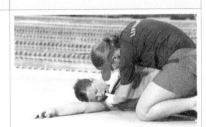
4	Measure the suction tip. • Measure from the angle of the person's jaw to the corner of the mouth. • Note the distance to avoid inserting the suction tip too deeply.	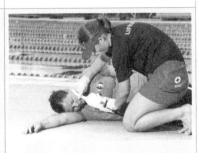

Continued

Using a Suctioning Device (Continued)

5	Check that the suction is working. • **Manual device:** Place your gloved finger over the end of the suction tip as you squeeze the handle of the device. • **Mechanical device:** Turn the unit on and follow the manufacturer's directions for checking that that the suction is working.	
6	Suction the mouth. • Insert the suction tip into the back of the mouth. • Apply suction as you withdraw the catheter using a sweeping motion, if possible. • If using a manual device, squeeze the handle repeatedly to apply suction. • Suction for **no more than:** • **Adult:** 15 seconds at a time • **Child:** 10 seconds at a time • **Infant:** 5 seconds at a time	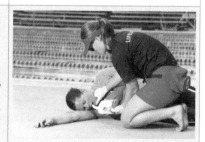

Skill Sheet 3-4. **Administering Emergency Oxygen— Variable-Flow-Rate System**

1	Check the cylinder. • Make sure that the oxygen cylinder is labeled "U.S.P." (United States Pharmacopeia) and marked with a yellow diamond that says "Oxygen."	
2	Clear the valve. • Remove the protective covering. • Remove and save the O-ring gasket, if present. • Turn the cylinder away from you and others before opening the cylinder valve. • Open the cylinder valve for 1 second to clear the valve of any debris.	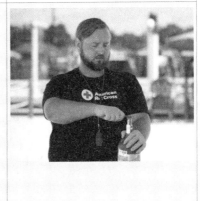

Continued

3	Attach the pressure regulator. • If you removed the O-ring gasket, put it into the valve on the top of the cylinder. • Make sure the pressure regulator is designed for delivering emergency oxygen and that the O-ring gasket is secure. • Check to see that the pin index on the pressure regulator corresponds to the oxygen cylinder. • Secure the pressure regulator on the cylinder by placing the two metal prongs into the valve. • Hand-tighten the screw until the regulator is snug.	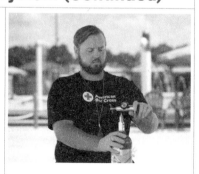
4	Open the cylinder counterclockwise one full turn. • Check the pressure gauge to verify that the cylinder has enough pressure (more than 200 psi). **NOTE!** If the pressure is lower than 200 psi, do not use the cylinder.	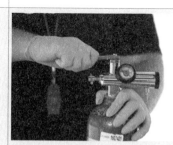

Continued

Administering Emergency Oxygen—Variable-Flow-Rate System (Continued)

5	Attach the delivery device. • Attach the plastic tubing between the pressure regulator and the delivery device.	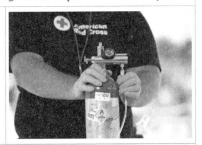
6	Turn the flowmeter to the desired flow rate. • **Nasal cannula:** 1 to 6 LPM • **Simple oxygen face mask:** 6 to 15 LPM • **Nonrebreather mask:** 10 to 15 LPM • **BVM resuscitator:** ≥ 15 LPM	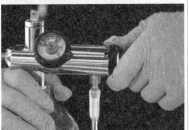
7	Verify the oxygen flow. • When using a nonrebreather mask or BVM resuscitator, ensure that the oxygen reservoir bag is two-thirds inflated by placing your thumb over the one-way valve. • Listen for a hissing sound and feel for oxygen flow through the delivery device.	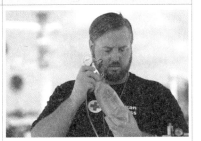

Continued

8	Place the delivery device on the person.	
9	Continue care until EMS professionals arrive and take over.	
10	Break down the oxygen delivery system. • Reverse the assembly steps. • Bleed the pressure regulator by turning on the flowmeter after the cylinder has been turned off.	

Skill Sheet 3-5. **Obstructed Airway Care— Adult/Child**

NOTE! Back blows, abdominal thrusts and chest thrusts are all equally effective, but it may take more than one technique to clear the airway. Additionally, in some situations it may be appropriate to give chest thrusts instead of abdominal thrusts.

| 1 | Recognize an airway obstruction.

• If the person is able to speak to you or is coughing forcefully, they may have a partial airway obstruction.
  • Encourage them to keep coughing but be prepared to intervene if their condition changes.
  • Reassess the person, recognize issues, and provide care as needed.

• If the person is unable to speak to you or is coughing weakly, they may have a complete airway obstruction.
  • Immediately instruct someone to call 9-1-1 and get the equipment.
  • Provide care as noted below. | |

Continued

2	Obtain consent.	
	• **Adult:** Obtain consent from the person. • **Child:** Obtain consent from the parent or legal guardian if present. If they are not available, consent is implied.	

3	Give 5 back blows.
	
	• Position yourself to the side and slightly behind the person.
	  • If the person is a young child or in a wheelchair, you may need to kneel.
	
	• Place one arm diagonally across the person's chest and bend them forward at the waist.
	  • The person's upper body should be as parallel to the ground as possible.
	
	• Using the heel of your other hand, give 5 firm back blows between the person's shoulder blades.
	  • Make each back blow a separate and distinct attempt to dislodge the object.
		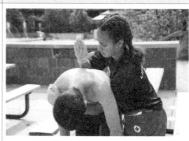
		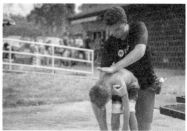

Continued

4A Give 5 abdominal thrusts.

• Use one or two fingers to find the person's navel.

• Move behind the person and place your front foot in between the person's feet with your knees slightly bent to provide balance and stability.
  • If the person is a young child or in a wheelchair, you may need to kneel.

• Make a fist with your other hand and place the thumb side against the person's abdomen, right above your fingers.

• Cover your fist with your other hand.

• Pull inward and upward to give an abdominal thrust.
  • Make each abdominal thrust a separate and distinct attempt to dislodge the object.

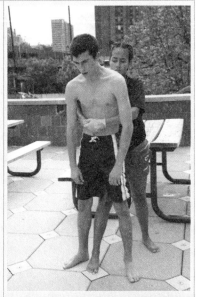

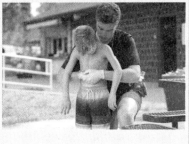

Continued

4B	Give 5 chest thrusts.	
	• Position yourself behind the person as you would for abdominal thrusts.	
	• If the person is a young child or in a wheelchair, you may need to kneel.	
	• Place the thumb side of your fist against the center of the person's chest on the lower half of the sternum.	
	• Cover your fist with your other hand.	
	• Pull straight back to give a chest thrust.	
	• Make each chest thrust a separate and distinct attempt to dislodge the object.	
5	Continue giving sets of 5 back blows and 5 abdominal thrusts (or chest thrusts) until:	
	• The person can cough forcefully, speak, cry or breathe.	
	• The person becomes unresponsive.	

Continued

6 | If the person becomes unresponsive:

• Ensure they are on a firm, flat surface and immediately begin CPR, starting with compressions.
  • **Single-rescuer CPR:** 30:2 (adult and child)
  • **Multiple-rescuer CPR:** 30:2 (adult), 15:2 (child)

• After each set of compressions and before attempting ventilations, open the person's mouth, look for the object, and, if seen, remove it with a finger sweep.

NOTE! Never do a finger sweep unless you actually see the object.

NOTE! Never attempt more than 2 ventilations during one cycle of CPR even if the chest does not rise.

Obstructed Airway Care— Infant

1	Recognize an airway obstruction.	

	• If the infant is crying or coughing forcefully, they may have a partial airway obstruction.
	   • Allow the infant to keep coughing but be prepared to intervene if their condition changes.
	   • Reassess the infant, recognize issues, and provide care as needed.
	
	 • If the infant is unable to cry or is coughing weakly, they may have a complete airway obstruction.
	   • Immediately instruct someone to call 9-1-1 and get emergency equipment.
	   • Provide care as noted below.	

2	Obtain consent from the parent or legal guardian if present. If they are not available, consent is implied.	

Continued

3 | Give 5 back blows.

- Place your forearm along the infant's back, cradling the back of the infant's head with your hand.

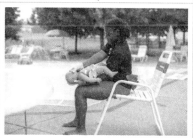

- Place your other forearm along the infant's front, supporting the infant's jaw with your thumb and fingers.
  - Do not cover the infant's face.

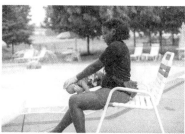

- Turn the infant face-down.
  - Hold them along your forearm and use your thigh for support.
  - Keep the infant's head lower than their body.

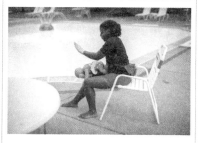

- Use the heel of your hand to give a back blow between the infant's shoulder blades.
  - Keep your fingers up to avoid hitting the infant's head or neck.
  - Make each back blow a separate and distinct attempt to dislodge the object.

Continued

Skill Sheet 3-6. **Obstructed Airway Care— Infant (Continued)**

4	Give 5 chest thrusts. • Position the infant between your forearms. • Support the head and neck. • Turn the infant face-up. • Lower the infant onto your thigh with their head lower than their chest. • Place two fingers in the center of the infant's chest, just below the nipple line. • Give 5 quick chest thrusts about 1½ inches deep. • Let the chest return to its normal position, keeping your fingers in contact with the breastbone. • Make each chest thrust a separate and distinct attempt to dislodge the object.	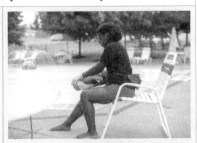 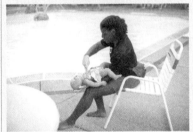
5	Continue giving sets of 5 back blows and 5 chest thrusts until: • The infant can cough forcefully, cry or breathe. • The infant becomes unresponsive.	

Continued

6 If the infant becomes unresponsive:

- Ensure they are on a firm, flat surface and immediately begin CPR, starting with compressions.
  - **Single-rescuer CPR:** 30:2
  - **Multiple-rescuer CPR:** 15:2
- After each set of compressions and before attempting ventilations, open the infant's mouth, look for the object, and, if seen, remove it with a finger sweep using your pinky finger.

NOTE! Never do a finger sweep unless you actually see the object.

NOTE! Never attempt more than 2 ventilations during one cycle of CPR even if the chest does not rise.

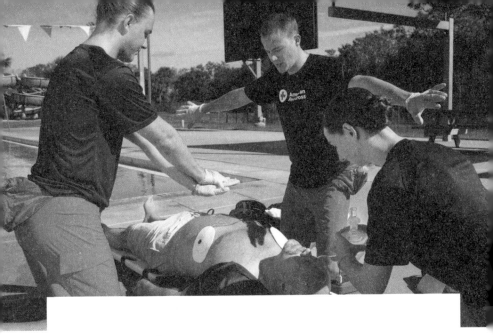

CPR AND AED

Cardiac arrest can happen at any time to a person of any age. When a person experiences cardiac arrest, quick action on the part of those who witness the arrest is crucial. Recognizing cardiac arrest and activating the emergency medical services (EMS) system, providing high-quality CPR and using an AED as soon as one is available gives the person the greatest chance for survival.

4:1 CARDIAC ARREST

Cardiac arrest occurs when the heart stops beating or beats too ineffectively to circulate blood to the brain and other vital organs. Causes of cardiac arrest include:

+ Drowning and other breathing emergencies.

+ Cardiovascular emergencies, such as a heart attack (myocardial infarction).

+ Electrocution.

+ Trauma.

+ Toxicity, such as from a drug overdose or poisoning.

Cardiac arrest frequently happens suddenly and without any warning signs or symptoms. When this occurs, the person is said to have experienced **sudden cardiac arrest**. People who have a history of cardiovascular disease or a congenital heart condition are at higher risk for sudden cardiac arrest, but sudden cardiac arrest can also occur in people who appear healthy and have no known heart disease or other risk factors.

You may see a person who is experiencing cardiac arrest suddenly collapse. When you check for responsiveness, breathing and a pulse during your rapid assessment, you will find that the person is not responsive, not breathing (or only gasping) and has no pulse.

 THE PROS KNOW

Agonal breaths (isolated or infrequent gasping in the absence of normal breathing) can occur even after the heart has stopped beating and may be seen early in cardiac arrest. Do not mistake agonal breaths for normal breathing.

4:2 THE CARDIAC CHAIN OF SURVIVAL

The Cardiac Chain of Survival describes six actions that, when performed in rapid succession, increase the person's likelihood of surviving cardiac arrest and recovering. Each link in the chain depends on, and is interconnected to, the other links. There is a Cardiac Chain of Survival for adults and one for children and infants.

The six links in the Adult Cardiac Chain of Survival (Figure 4-1A) are:

+ **Recognition of a cardiac emergency and activation of the emergency response system.** Immediate recognition of cardiac arrest and activation of the EMS system provides the person with access to necessary personnel, equipment and interventions as soon after arrest as possible.

+ **Early high-quality CPR.** High-quality CPR should be initiated immediately once cardiac arrest is recognized, ideally by those at the scene prior to EMS arrival.

+ **Early defibrillation.** Use of an AED by those at the scene prior to EMS arrival may restore an effective heart rhythm, increasing the person's chances for survival.

+ **Advanced life support.** Early advanced life support provided by EMS professionals at the scene and en route to the hospital provides the person with access to emergency medical care delivered by trained professionals.

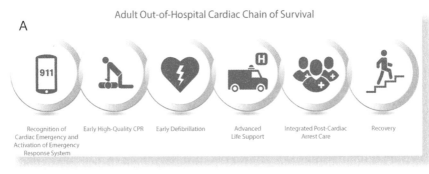

Adult Out-of-Hospital Cardiac Chain of Survival

A

| Recognition of Cardiac Emergency and Activation of Emergency Response System | Early High-Quality CPR | Early Defibrillation | Advanced Life Support | Integrated Post-Cardiac Arrest Care | Recovery |

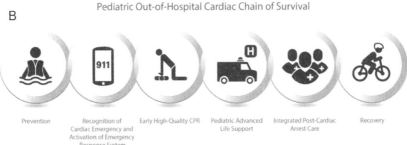

Pediatric Out-of-Hospital Cardiac Chain of Survival

B

| Prevention | Recognition of Cardiac Emergency and Activation of Emergency Response System | Early High-Quality CPR | Pediatric Advanced Life Support | Integrated Post-Cardiac Arrest Care | Recovery |

Figure 4-1 Professional rescuers and other team members play a major role in completing actions in the Cardiac Chains of Survival. **(A)** Adult Cardiac Chain of Survival. **(B)** Pediatric Cardiac Chain of Survival.

+ **Integrated post-cardiac arrest care.** After the person is resuscitated, survival outcomes are improved when an interdisciplinary team of medical professionals works to stabilize the person's medical condition, minimize complications, and diagnose and treat the underlying cause of the cardiac arrest.

+ **Recovery.** After the person is discharged from the hospital, continued follow-up during the recovery process in the form of rehabilitation, therapy, and support from family and healthcare providers improves outcomes.

The Pediatric Cardiac Chain of Survival is slightly different from the Adult Cardiac Chain of Survival (Figure 4-1B). Because cardiac arrest in children and infants most often occurs as the result of a preventable injury (such as drowning), **prevention** is the first link in the Pediatric Cardiac Chain of Survival. The second link is **recognition of the cardiac emergency and activation of the emergency response system**, and the third link is **early high-quality CPR.** The fourth link is **pediatric advanced life support,** and, just as in the Adult Cardiac Chain of Survival, the last two links are **integrated post-cardiac arrest care** and **recovery**.

Professional rescuers and other team members play a vital role in implementing the first three links in both the Adult and Pediatric Cardiac Chains of Survival. When you recognize that a person is in cardiac arrest, you must act quickly. Instruct another team member to call EMS and get resuscitation equipment, including an AED. Begin CPR immediately and use an AED as soon as possible.

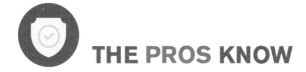

THE PROS KNOW

For each minute that CPR and use of an AED are delayed, a person's chance for survival decreases by 7 to 10 percent.

Although the principles of providing CPR and using an AED are the same for people of all ages, there are some differences in technique and equipment that you need to consider for children and infants. Box 4-1 provides definitions to help you determine whether a person is an infant, a child or an adolescent and summarizes age-dependent CPR/AED guidelines.

Box 4-1 CPR/AED GUIDELINES

CPR Guidelines

When providing CPR, you need to know whether a person is an infant, a child or an adolescent.

	Definition	CPR Guideline
	An **infant** is defined as a person younger than 1 year.	Follow **infant** techniques and use appropriately sized equipment.
	A **child** is defined as a person from the age of 1 year to the onset of puberty, as evidenced by breast development in girls and underarm hair development in boys (usually around the age of 12 years).	Follow **child** techniques and use appropriately sized equipment.
	An **adolescent** is defined as a person from the onset of puberty to adulthood.	Follow **adult** techniques and use appropriately sized equipment.

Continued

Box 4-1 CPR/AED GUIDELINES (Continued)

AED Guidelines

AED guidelines are based on the person's age and weight, rather than on developmental stage. Some AEDs come with pediatric AED pads that are smaller and designed specifically to analyze a child's heart rhythm and deliver a lower level of energy. Other AEDs have a key or a switch that configures the AED to deliver a lower level of energy for use on a person who is younger than 8 years or who weighs less than 55 pounds (25 kilograms).

For children **up to 8 years of age** (including infants) or **weighing less than 55 pounds** (25 kilograms), use **pediatric AED pads** and the **pediatric setting** on the AED if they are available. If pediatric AED pads and a pediatric setting are not available, it is safe to use adult AED pads and the adult setting.

For children **older than 8 years of age** (including adolescents) or **weighing more than 55 pounds** (25 kilograms), use **adult AED pads** and the **adult setting** on the AED. Do not use pediatric AED pads or the pediatric setting because the shock delivered will not be sufficient.

4:3 CPR

The objective of CPR is to circulate oxygenated blood to vital organs when the heart and normal breathing have stopped. CPR consists of chest compressions and ventilations, delivered in cycles. Even when performed perfectly, CPR provides only a fraction of the normal blood flow to the brain and heart. Providing high-quality CPR (Box 4-2) optimizes outcomes and increases the likelihood of **return of spontaneous circulation (ROSC)** (successful resuscitation, evidenced by the return of a regular heart rhythm capable of sustaining adequate blood flow throughout the body).

When you are working as a professional rescuer, you may need to provide single-rescuer CPR before other team members arrive to help. In **single-rescuer CPR**, the rescuer transitions between giving

Box 4-2 HIGH-QUALITY CPR

To provide high-quality CPR, follow these key principles.

+ Position the person on their back on a **firm, flat surface** and expose their chest, then immediately begin chest compressions.

+ Provide **compressions** at the **correct rate** and at the **proper depth.**

	Rate	Depth
Adult	100 to 120 per minute	At least 2 inches
Child	100 to 120 per minute	About 2 inches
Infant	100 to 120 per minute	About 1½ inches

+ **Allow for full chest recoil.** Allowing the chest to return to its normal position after each compression allows the heart to fill adequately, maximizing the amount of blood that is sent out to the rest of the body with the next compression.

+ **Minimize necessary interruptions to chest compressions.** When compressions stop, blood flow to vital organs stops. When you must briefly stop compressions (for example, to give ventilations or deliver a shock using an AED), keep the interruption to less than 10 seconds. The **chest compression fraction (CCF)** represents the amount of time spent performing compressions and can be used as a measure of high-quality CPR. It is calculated by dividing the time that rescuers are in contact with the person's chest by the total duration of the resuscitation event, beginning with the arrival of the resuscitation team and ending with the achievement of return of spontaneous circulation (ROSC) or the cessation of CPR. According to expert consensus, a CCF of at least 60% is needed to promote optimal outcomes, and the goal should be 80%.

+ **Avoid excessive ventilations.** Each ventilation should last about 1 second and deliver just enough volume to make the chest begin to rise.

Continued

sets of chest compressions and ventilations (Figure 4-2). When an additional rescuer who is trained in CPR is available, you should provide **two-rescuer CPR**. In two-rescuer CPR, one rescuer gives chest compressions and the other gives ventilations (Figure 4-3), and the rescuers switch roles at least every 2 minutes (or whenever the rescuer giving compressions indicates that they are tiring). This helps to minimize rescuer fatigue, which in turn helps to maintain the quality of compressions and supports the delivery of high-quality CPR.

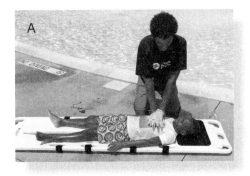

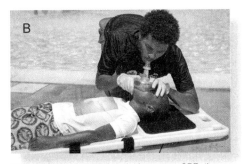

Compressions

Using proper technique when providing compressions is essential for providing high-quality CPR.

Figure 4-2 When providing single-rescuer CPR, the same rescuer gives **(A)** chest compressions and **(B)** ventilations.

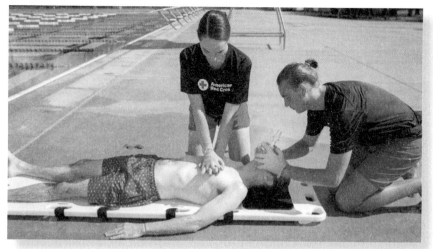

Figure 4-3 During two-rescuer CPR, one rescuer gives chest compressions and the other rescuer gives ventilations.

Adult or Child

First, make sure the person is lying face-up on a firm, flat surface. If the person is on a soft surface, quickly and carefully move them to the ground before you begin. Kneel beside the person's chest with your knees near their body. Spread your knees about shoulder-width apart.

Position the heel of one hand in the center of the chest on the person's sternum (breastbone). If you feel the notch at the end of the sternum, move your hand slightly toward the person's head. Place your other hand on top of your first hand and interlace your fingers or hold them up so that your fingers are not on the person's chest. Position yourself so that your shoulders are directly over your hands and lock your elbows to keep your arms straight (Figure 4-4). Compress the chest using a straight down-and-up motion. This motion moves the most blood with each compression and is less tiring for the rescuer.

Push straight down (*at least* 2 inches in an adult and *about* 2 inches in a child), and then let the chest recoil (return to its normal position). Keep your hands on the person's chest, but avoid leaning. Push hard and push fast! You want to give compressions at a rate of 100 to 120 compressions per minute, or about one compression every half second. As you give compressions, count each one out loud. In most cases, compressions

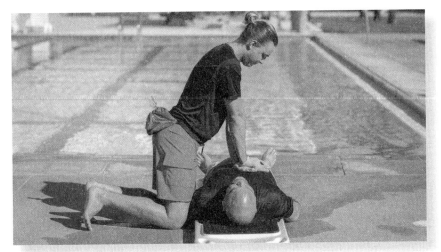

Figure 4-4 Proper technique is essential when giving compressions. Position your body so that your shoulders are directly over your hands and lock your elbows to keep your arms straight.

are given in sets of 30. Maintain a smooth, steady down-and-up rhythm and do not pause between compressions.

For a smaller child, you may use one hand instead of two hands to give compressions (Figure 4-5). When using one hand, be sure you are able to compress the chest about 2 inches. Simply place the heel of one hand in the center of the chest and give compressions.

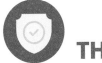 **THE PROS KNOW**

Incorrect technique or body position can cause your arms and shoulders to tire quickly when you are giving compressions. Use the weight of your upper body, not your arm muscles, to compress the chest. Avoid rocking back and forth. Rocking makes your compressions less effective and wastes energy. Keep your hands on the person's chest, but avoid leaning. Leaning prevents the chest from returning to its normal position after each compression, which limits the amount of blood that can return to the heart. This, in turn, limits the amount of blood that can be delivered to the rest of the body with the next compression.

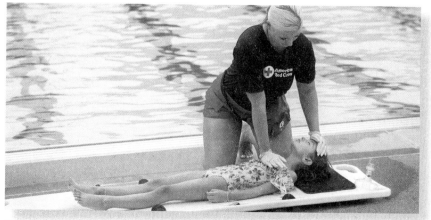

Figure 4-5 For a small child, you can use one hand to give compressions.

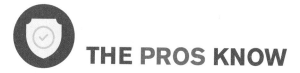

THE PROS KNOW

Counting out loud as you give compressions helps you to keep a steady, even rhythm and helps other rescuers anticipate a switch from compressions to ventilations or a role change. To call for a role change, say "switch" in place of the number "1" at the beginning of the CPR cycle.

Infant

The general principles of giving compressions to an infant are the same as for an adult or child, but the technique is different because of the infant's smaller size. As with an adult or child, first make sure the infant is on a firm, flat surface and expose the infant's chest. Then, use the encircling thumbs technique (Figure 4-6A) to give compressions. When you are providing single-rescuer CPR, you may use the two-finger technique (Figure 4-6B) instead of the encircling thumbs technique to give compressions. If the required depth for compressions cannot be achieved using either technique, you may consider using a one-hand technique similar to what you would use for a small child.

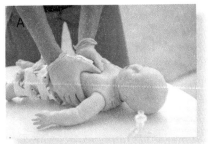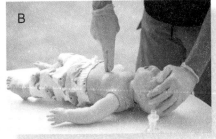

Figure 4-6 To provide compressions to an infant, use **(A)** the encircling thumbs technique or **(B)** the two-finger technique.

Encircling thumbs technique

Stand or kneel to the side of the infant with your hips at a slight angle. Place both of your thumbs side by side on the center of the infant's chest, just below the nipple line, and wrap your remaining fingers around the infant's torso, providing support (see Figure 4-6A). Using both thumbs at the same time, compress the chest about 1½ inches at a rate of 100 to 120 compressions per minute. As you give compressions, count each one out loud. Maintain a smooth, steady down-and-up rhythm and do not pause between compressions. Let the chest return to its normal position after each compression.

Two-finger technique

When using the two-finger technique, you can use your index and middle fingers or your middle and fourth fingers. Fingers that are more similar in length tend to make compressions easier to perform.

Stand or kneel to the side of the infant and, using your hand that is closest to the infant's feet, place two fingers in the center of the chest, just below the nipple line (see Figure 4-6B). If you feel the notch at the end of the infant's sternum, move your fingers slightly toward the infant's head. The fingers should be oriented so that they are parallel, not perpendicular to, the sternum. Place your other hand on the infant's forehead to help keep the airway open while you give compressions. Using both fingers at the same time, compress the chest about 1½ inches at a rate of 100 to 120 compressions per minute. As you give compressions, count each one out loud. Maintain a smooth, steady down-and-up rhythm and do not pause between compressions. Let the chest return to its normal position after each compression.

Ventilations

After each set of compressions, give 2 ventilations. Give 1 ventilation, pause briefly to allow the person's chest to fall, then give another ventilation. If the chest does not rise after the first ventilation, reopen the airway, make a seal and try another ventilation. Never attempt more than 2 ventilations before resuming compressions. The process of giving 2 ventilations and then resuming compressions should take less than 10 seconds.

Remember that when you are giving ventilations to a person during CPR, you should:

+ Smoothly transition between giving chest compressions and giving ventilations.

+ Use a resuscitation mask or— if three or more rescuers are available—a bag-valve-mask (BVM) resuscitator.

+ Maintain an open airway using the head-tilt/chin-lift technique, the jaw-thrust maneuver with head extension or the modified jaw-thrust maneuver.

+ Position and seal the mask properly over the person's mouth and nose.

+ Avoid excessive ventilation. Each ventilation should last about 1 second and make the person's chest begin to rise. Allow the person's chest to fall before delivering the next ventilation.

ⓘ CARE ALERT

During CPR, the person may vomit. If this occurs, quickly turn the person onto their side to prevent the vomit from blocking the airway and entering the lungs. Clear the person's airway using a gloved finger and, if one is available and you are trained to use it, a suctioning device. Then roll the person onto their back and continue giving care.

CPR Cycles

In most cases, CPR is provided in cycles of 30 chest compressions followed by 2 ventilations. However, because the cause of cardiac arrest in children and infants is most often a breathing emergency (such as drowning), you should provide cycles of 15 compressions followed by 2 ventilations when the person is a child or infant *and* two or more rescuers are available to perform CPR. This provides more frequent ventilations for children and infants while minimizing interruptions to compressions. Table 4-1 summarizes CPR technique for adults, children and infants.

Table 4-1. Comparison of CPR Technique in Adults, Children and Infants

Adult	Child	Infant
About 12 years or older	Between the ages of 1 and 12 years	Younger than 1 year
Positioning		
• Kneel beside the person. • Two hands in center of chest; fingers interlaced and off the chest • Shoulders directly over hands; elbows locked	• Kneel beside the person. • Two hands in center of chest; fingers interlaced and off the chest • Shoulders directly over hands; elbows locked	• Stand or kneel to the side of the infant, with your hips slightly angled. • Both thumbs (side-by-side) on the center of the infant's chest, just below the nipple line • Fingers encircle the infant's torso, providing support
	Note: Alternatively, you can use the one-hand technique.	**Note:** Alternatively, when providing single-rescuer CPR, you can use the two-finger technique or the one-hand technique.

Continued

Table 4-1. Comparison of CPR Technique in Adults, Children and Infants (Continued)

Adult	Child	Infant
Compressions		
• Push hard and fast. • Compress *at least 2 inches.* • Rate: 100 to 120 compressions per minute	• Push hard and fast. • Compress *about 2 inches.* • Rate: 100 to 120 compressions per minute	• Push hard and fast. • Compress *about 1½ inches.* • Rate: 100 to 120 compressions per minute
Ventilations		
• Seal the mask over the mouth and nose and open the airway to a **past-neutral position.**	• Seal the mask over the mouth and nose and open the airway to a **slightly past-neutral position.**	• Seal the mask over the mouth and nose and open the airway to **neutral position.**
Cycles		
• **One-rescuer CPR:** 30 chest compressions and 2 ventilations **(30:2)** • **Two-rescuer CPR:** 30 chest compressions and 2 ventilations **(30:2)**	• **One-rescuer CPR:** 30 chest compressions and 2 ventilations **(30:2)** • **Two-rescuer CPR:** 15 chest compressions and 2 ventilations **(15:2)**	• **One-rescuer CPR:** 30 chest compressions and 2 ventilations **(30:2)** • **Two-rescuer CPR:** 15 chest compressions and 2 ventilations **(15:2)**

Once you begin CPR, continue giving cycles of chest compressions and ventilations. Continue cycles of CPR until:

+ You see signs of ROSC, such as movement, breathing or coughing.

+ An AED is ready to analyze the heart rhythm.

+ Other trained providers take over and relieve you from giving compressions and ventilations.

+ You are too exhausted to continue.

+ The situation becomes unsafe.

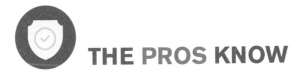

THE PROS KNOW

Many people who experience cardiac arrest do not survive. Participating in a resuscitation effort, even a successful one, can have a psychological impact on rescuers. Mental health treatment provided by a qualified mental health professional can be beneficial following a resuscitation or other stressful event.

Skill Sheets 4-1 and 4-2 provide step-by-step instructions for adult/child single-rescuer CPR and infant single-rescuer CPR, respectively. Skill Sheets 4-3 and 4-4 provide step-by-step instructions for adult/child two-rescuer CPR and for infant two-rescuer CPR, respectively.

4:4 AED

While CPR can help to prevent brain damage and death by keeping oxygenated blood moving throughout the body, an AED can correct the underlying problem for some people who go into sudden cardiac arrest (Figure 4-7). Two abnormal heart rhythms in particular, **ventricular**

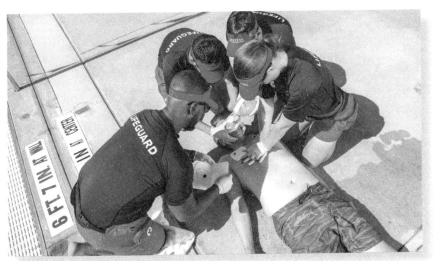

Figure 4-7 When a person is in cardiac arrest, providing CPR and using an AED as soon as one is available is critical.

fibrillation (V-fib) and **ventricular tachycardia (V-tach)**, can lead to sudden cardiac arrest. In ventricular fibrillation, the heart muscle simply quivers (fibrillates) weakly instead of contracting strongly. In ventricular tachycardia, the heart muscle contracts too fast (*tachy-* means "fast"). Both abnormal rhythms impair the heart's ability to pump and circulate blood throughout the body and are life-threatening. However, in many cases, ventricular fibrillation and ventricular tachycardia can be corrected by an electrical shock delivered by an AED. This shock disrupts the heart's electrical activity long enough to allow the heart to spontaneously develop an effective rhythm on its own. Not all abnormal heart rhythms seen in cardiac arrest are shockable, however. The AED analyzes the heart's rhythm and, if it detects a shockable rhythm (ventricular fibrillation or ventricular tachycardia), it advises the rescuer to deliver a shock.

Different types of AEDs are available, but all are similar in their operation and use visual displays, voice prompts, or both to guide the rescuer. As a professional rescuer, you must know where the AED is located and how to operate it. You may also be responsible for ensuring that the AED is in good working order and ready for use (Box 4-3). Taking note of the locations of AEDs in public places that you frequent, such as shopping centers, airports, recreation centers and sports arenas, is also a good habit to develop.

Box 4-3 AED MAINTENANCE

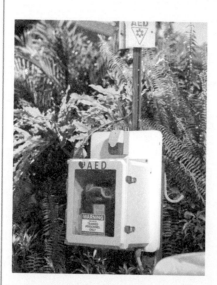

AEDs require minimal maintenance, but it is important to check them regularly according to the manufacturer's instructions or your employer's policy to ensure they are in good working order and ready for use whenever they are needed.

+ Familiarize yourself with the method the AED uses to indicate the status of

Continued

Box 4-3 AED MAINTENANCE (Continued)

the device. Many AEDs have a status indicator that displays a symbol or illuminates to indicate that the AED is in proper working order and ready to respond. The status indicator may also display symbols indicating that routine maintenance (for example, a battery change) is needed or that a problem with the device has been detected. Some AEDs have a warning indicator that will illuminate or beep if the AED is not in proper working order and ready to respond.

+ Check to make sure the battery is properly installed and within its expiration date.

+ Make sure AED pads are adequately stocked, stored in a sealed package and within their expiration date.

+ After using the AED, make sure that all supplies are restocked and that the device is in proper working order.

+ If at any time the AED fails to work properly or warning indicators illuminate, take the AED out of service and contact the manufacturer or the appropriate person at your facility, according to your employer's policy. You may need to return the AED to the manufacturer for service. If the AED stops working during an emergency, continue giving CPR until EMS personnel arrive and begin their care of the person.

+ Team members who are responsible for maintaining the AED should familiarize themselves with the owner's manual and follow the manufacturer's instructions for maintaining the equipment.

Using an AED

To use an AED, first turn the device on. Remove or cut away clothing and undergarments to expose the person's chest. If the person's chest is wet, dry it using a towel or a gauze pad (Figure 4-8). Dry skin helps the AED pads to stick properly. Do not use an alcohol wipe to dry the skin because alcohol is flammable and could burn the person's skin if a shock is delivered.

Next, place the AED pads. Always use adult AED pads on any person who is 8 years or older and/or weighs more than 55 pounds (25 kilograms). If the person is younger than 8 years or weighs less than 55 pounds (25 kilograms), use pediatric AED pads or settings if you have them, but if all you have is an AED with adult pads or adult settings, use the adult pads or settings.

ⓘ CARE ALERT

If pediatric AED pads or a pediatric setting are not available, it is safe to use adult AED pads or the adult setting on a person who is younger than 8 years and/or who weighs less than 55 pounds (25 kilograms). However, the reverse is not true! Do not use pediatric AED pads or a pediatric setting on a person who is older than 8 years and/or who weighs more than 55 pounds (25 kilograms). For these people, the shock delivered will not be sufficient if pediatric pads or the pediatric setting are used.

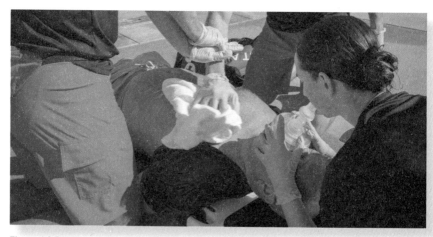

Figure 4-8 Dry the person's chest using a towel or gauze pad before applying the AED pads.

Peel the backing off the pads as directed, one at a time, to expose the adhesive. Place one pad on the upper right side of the person's chest and the other pad on the lower left side of the person's chest, a few inches below the left armpit, pressing firmly to adhere (Figure 4-9). Make sure the AED pads do not touch each other when they are applied to the chest. If you cannot position the pads on the chest without them touching (for example,

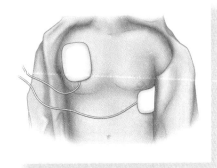

Figure 4-9 Place one AED pad on the upper right side of the chest and the other on the lower left side of the chest, below the person's left armpit.

on an infant or a small child), position one pad in the middle of the chest and the other pad on the back between the shoulder blades (Figure 4-10).

Plug the pad connector cable into the AED (if necessary) and follow the device's directions. Most AEDs will begin to analyze the heart rhythm automatically, but some may require you to push an "analyze" button to start this process. No one should touch the person while the AED is analyzing the heart rhythm because this could result in a faulty reading. Say "CLEAR!" in a loud, commanding voice and be ready to deliver a shock if the AED determines one is needed. Next, the AED will tell you to push the "shock" button if a shock is advised. Again, avoid touching the person, because anyone who is touching the person while the device is delivering a shock is at risk for receiving a shock as well. Say "CLEAR!" in a loud, commanding voice and, if a shock is advised, push the shock button to deliver the shock.

After a shock is delivered (or if the AED determines no shock is necessary), immediately resume CPR, beginning with compressions. The AED will continue to check the heart rhythm every 2 minutes. Listen for prompts from the AED. Continue giving CPR until:

+ The AED prompts that it is reanalyzing.

+ You see signs of ROSC, such as movement, breathing or coughing.

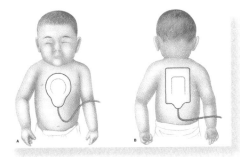

Figure 4-10 For an infant, or if the pads risk touching each other when placed on the chest of a small child, place one pad on the middle of the chest and the other pad on the back between the shoulder blades.

+ Other trained providers take over and relieve you from giving compressions and ventilations.

+ You are too exhausted to continue.

+ The situation becomes unsafe.

When a person is in cardiac arrest, use an AED as soon as possible. If CPR is in progress when the AED arrives, do not interrupt chest compressions and ventilations until the AED is turned on, the AED pads are applied and the AED is ready to analyze the heart rhythm, unless you are the only rescuer trained to operate the AED and provide CPR. When two trained rescuers are available, the steps for using an AED are the same, but one rescuer performs CPR while the other operates the AED (Figure 4-11). The two rescuers switch roles about every 2 minutes, or as the AED is analyzing the heart rhythm, to minimize rescuer fatigue and support the delivery of high-quality CPR.

Environmental and person-specific considerations for safe and effective AED use are given in Box 4-4.

Skill Sheet 4-5 provides step-by-step instructions for using an AED.

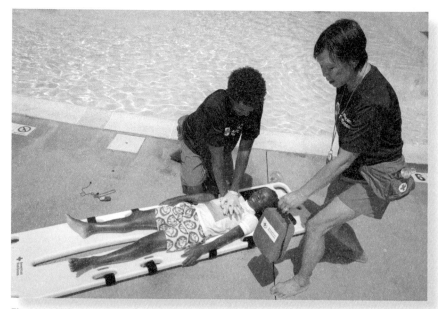

Figure 4-11 When two trained rescuers are available, one rescuer performs CPR while the other operates the AED, and they switch roles about every 2 minutes.

Box 4-4 CONSIDERATIONS FOR SAFE AND EFFECTIVE AED USE

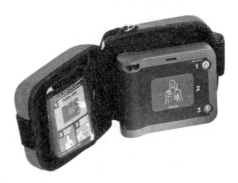

Environmental Considerations

+ **Water.** If the person is in the water, extricate them before using the AED. Once you have removed them from the water, be sure there are no deep puddles of water around you, the person or the AED. Avoid getting the AED or the AED pads wet. Remove wet clothing and wipe the person's chest dry before applying the AED pads.

+ **Inclement weather.** It is safe to use AEDs in all weather conditions, including rain and snow. Provide a dry environment if possible (for example, by sheltering the person with umbrellas), but do not delay administering a shock to do so. Avoid getting the AED or the AED pads wet. Remove wet clothing and wipe the person's chest dry before applying the AED pads.

+ **Metal surfaces.** It is safe to use an AED when the person is lying on a metal surface, as long as appropriate precautions are taken. Do not allow the AED pads to contact the metal surface, and ensure that no one is touching the person when the shock is delivered.

+ **Flammable or combustible materials.** Do not use an AED around flammable or combustible materials, such as gasoline or free-flowing oxygen. If oxygen is being administered to a person when the AED is ready to be used, make sure to close the tank before shocking.

Continued

Box 4-4 CONSIDERATIONS FOR SAFE AND EFFECTIVE AED USE (Continued)

Person-Specific Considerations

+ **Pregnancy.** It is safe to use an AED on a person who is pregnant.

+ **Trauma.** If a person is in cardiac arrest and has traumatic injuries, you should still use an AED.

+ **Hypothermia.** Do not delay CPR or use of an AED to rewarm the person. Remove wet clothing, dry the person's chest and protect the person from further heat loss while providing CPR and using the AED.

+ **Pacemakers and implantable cardioverter-defibrillators (ICDs).** A person who has a known arrhythmia (irregular heartbeat) may have a pacemaker or an ICD. These are small devices that are surgically implanted under the skin to automatically prevent or correct an irregular heartbeat. If the implanted device is visible or you know that the person has a pacemaker or ICD, adjust pad placement as necessary to avoid placing the AED pads directly over the device because doing so may interfere with the delivery of the shock. If you are not sure whether the person has an implanted device, place the pads as you normally would.

+ **Transdermal medication patches.** Some types of medications, including nitroglycerin (used to relieve chest pain caused by cardiovascular disease) and smoking cessation medications, are delivered through patches applied to the skin. Remove any medication patches that you see before applying AED pads and using an AED. Wear gloves to prevent absorption of the drug through your own skin.

+ **Chest hair.** Time is critical in a cardiac arrest situation and chest hair rarely interferes with pad adhesion, so in most cases, you

Continued

4:5 MULTIPLE-RESCUER TEAM RESPONSE

Care for an unresponsive person in cardiac arrest may begin with one rescuer, who performs the rapid assessment and begins CPR. When CPR is in progress with one rescuer, the second rescuer to arrive on the scene should confirm that EMS has been summoned. If EMS has not been summoned, the second rescuer to arrive on the scene should do so before getting the AED or assisting with care. As additional rescuers arrive on the scene, they join the team response and perform various roles as needed (Figure 4-12). When at least three rescuers are available, roles in a multiple-rescuer team response can include:

+ The **compressor,** who is responsible for chest compressions.

+ The **airway manager,** who is positioned behind the person's head and is responsible for placing and sealing the mask and maintaining an open airway.

+ The **ventilator,** who is responsible for squeezing the bag on the BVM resuscitator to deliver ventilations.

+ The **AED operator,** who is responsible for operating the AED.

①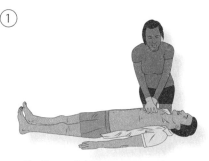

The first available rescuer completes the rapid assessment and begins CPR.

②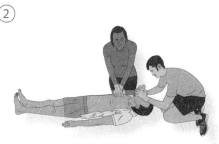

If available, two rescuers may perform two-rescuer CPR.

- One rescuer gives compressions ● while the other rescuer gives ventilations. ●
- The rescuers switch roles about every 2 minutes (5 cycles of 30:2).

③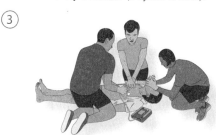

A rescuer uses the AED ● as soon as the AED is available.

- The rescuer(s) performing CPR continue providing compressions ● and ventilations ● until the AED pads are placed and the AED is ready to begin analyzing.

④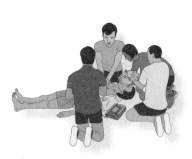

When two rescuers are available to operate the BVM resuscitator:

- One rescuer maintains the mask seal and an open airway. ●
- The other rescuer delivers ventilations. ●

⑤

The rescuers relieve the compressor about every 2 minutes or when the AED ● analyzes. The rescuers continue providing CPR ●●● until:

- The AED prompts that it is reanalyzing.
- They see signs of ROSC, such as movement, breathing or coughing.
- Other trained providers take over and relieve them from giving compressions and ventilations.
- They are too exhausted to continue.
- The situation becomes unsafe.

Figure 4-12 During a multiple-rescuer team response, every team member should be able to arrive on the scene and perform any of the roles necessary to provide proper care. This is one example of how rescuers can be integrated into the resuscitation effort as they arrive on the scene.

A multiple-rescuer team response contributes to the delivery of high-quality CPR and may improve outcomes by helping to minimize rescuer fatigue and interruptions to compressions. During the resuscitation effort, the rescuers should switch roles to relieve the compressor about every 2 minutes, or after about 5 cycles of 30 compressions and 2 ventilations.

To be most effective, a coordinated team response is needed. Critical thinking, decision-making and communication among team members are essential. You must be able to arrive on the scene, recognize what action needs to be taken and perform whatever role is needed. Every team member needs to be able to anticipate their own next actions, in addition to understanding and anticipating the next actions of other team members.

When participating in a multiple-rescuer team response, follow your employer's protocols, and always provide appropriate care for the conditions that you find. Use the AED as soon as it is available and ready to use. Using the AED takes priority over using a BVM resuscitator or administering emergency oxygen. If a rescuer is needed to get or prepare the AED, stop using the BVM resuscitator and provide two-rescuer CPR until the AED is ready to analyze.

4:6 WRAP-UP

Quick recognition of cardiac arrest and activation of the EMS system, along with the provision of high-quality CPR and use of an AED by rescuers at the scene, can be lifesaving. Because every minute counts when a person is experiencing cardiac arrest, the person's survival often depends on rescuers at the scene acting quickly and giving appropriate care until EMS professionals arrive and begin their care of the person. Effective and efficient teamwork is critical during the resuscitation effort and can increase the person's chances for survival.

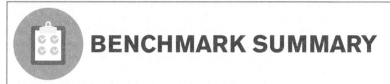

BENCHMARK SUMMARY

Benchmarks for Professional Rescuers

Professional rescuers should:

+ Strive to always provide high-quality CPR by:

  – Providing compressions at the correct rate and at the proper depth.

  – Allowing the chest to return to its normal position after each compression.

  – Minimizing necessary interruptions to chest compressions.

  – Avoiding excessive ventilations.

+ Be effective team members by:

  – Keeping their CPR/AED skills and knowledge current.

  – Using communication, critical thinking and decision-making skills.

  – Practicing working as part of a team to provide care for a person in cardiac arrest.

CPR—Single Rescuer (Adult/Child)

NOTE! Complete the rapid assessment and get an AED on the scene as soon as possible.

1	Ensure the person is on their back on a hard, flat surface. Kneel beside the person.

2   Give 30 chest compressions.

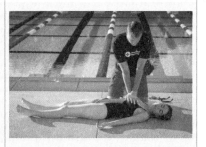

- Place the heel of one hand in the center of the person's chest with your other hand on top and your fingers interlaced and off the chest.

- Position your body so that your shoulders are directly over your hands; lock your elbows.

- Keeping your arms straight, push down, and then let the chest return to its normal position.
  - **Adult:** *at least* 2 inches
  - **Child:** *about* 2 inches

- Push hard and fast! Give compressions at a rate of 100 to 120 compressions per minute.

NOTE! Count out loud as you give compressions.

Continued

3	Give 2 ventilations.	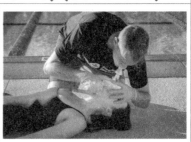

• Seal the mask and open the airway.
  • **Adult:** past-neutral position
  • **Child:** slightly past-neutral position

• Give 1 ventilation, pause briefly to allow the person's chest to fall, then give another ventilation.

• Each ventilation should last about 1 second and make the chest begin to rise.

NOTE! Minimize interruptions to chest compressions to **less than 10 seconds.**

NOTE! Never attempt more than 2 ventilations before resuming compressions. If the first ventilation does not cause the chest to rise, retilt the head and ensure a proper seal before giving the second ventilation. If the second ventilation does not make the chest rise, an object may be blocking the airway. Proceed with providing obstructed airway care for an unresponsive adult/child.

Continued

4	Continue giving cycles of 30 compressions and 2 ventilations until:
	• You see signs of ROSC, such as movement, breathing or coughing.
	• An AED is ready to analyze the heart rhythm.
	• Other trained providers take over and relieve you from giving compressions and ventilations.
	• You are too exhausted to continue.
	• The situation becomes unsafe.

CPR—Single Rescuer (Infant)

NOTE! Complete the rapid assessment and get an AED on the scene as soon as possible.

1	Ensure the infant is on their back on a hard, flat surface. Stand or kneel to the side of the infant, with your hips at a slight angle.
2	Give 30 chest compressions. 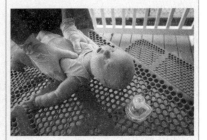

Step 2 continued:

- Place both thumbs (side-by-side) on the center of the infant's chest, just below the nipple line.

- Wrap your remaining fingers around the infant's torso, providing support.

- Using both thumbs at the same time, push down about 1½ inches, and then let the chest return to its normal position.

- Push hard and fast! Give compressions at a rate of 100 to 120 compressions per minute.

NOTE! Count out loud as you give compressions.

NOTE! Alternatively, you can use the two-finger technique. Stand or kneel to the side of the infant and give compressions using two fingers placed parallel to the sternum in the center of the chest.

CHAPTER 4: CPR AND AED

Continued

CPR—Single Rescuer (Infant) (Continued)

3	Give 2 ventilations.	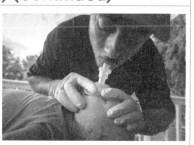

* Seal the mask and open the airway to a neutral position.

* Give 1 ventilation, pause briefly to allow the infant's chest to fall, then give another ventilation.

* Each ventilation should last about 1 second and make the chest begin to rise.

NOTE! Minimize interruptions to chest compressions to **less than 10 seconds.**

NOTE! Never attempt more than 2 ventilations before resuming compressions. If the first ventilation does not cause the chest to rise, retilt the head and ensure a proper seal before giving the second ventilation. If the second ventilation does not make the chest rise, an object may be blocking the airway. Proceed with providing obstructed airway care for an unresponsive infant.

Continued

4	Continue giving cycles of 30 compressions and 2 ventilations until:	
	• You see signs of ROSC, such as movement, breathing or coughing.	
	• An AED is ready to analyze the heart rhythm.	
	• Other trained providers take over and relieve you from giving compressions and ventilations.	
	• You are too exhausted to continue.	
	• The situation becomes unsafe.	

CPR—Two Rescuers (Adult/ Child)

NOTE! Complete the rapid assessment and get an AED on the scene as soon as possible.

1	Ensure the person is on their back on a hard, flat surface.
	
	• The rescuer providing compressions kneels beside the person.
	
	• The rescuer providing ventilations kneels above the person's head and prepares to give ventilations by sealing the mask and opening the airway.
	  • **Adult:** past-neutral position
	  • **Child:** slightly past-neutral position

2	The rescuer providing compressions gives chest compressions. • **Adult:** 30 compressions; compress to a depth of *at least* 2 inches • **Child:** 15 compressions; compress to a depth of *about* 2 inches • Push hard and fast! Give compressions at a rate of 100 to 120 compressions per minute. **NOTE:** Count out loud as you give compressions.

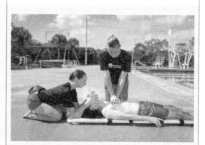

Continued

| 3 | The rescuer providing ventilations gives 2 ventilations. | 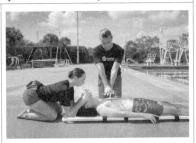 |

The rescuer providing ventilations gives 2 ventilations.

• Give 1 ventilation, pause briefly to allow the person's chest to fall, then give another ventilation.

• Each ventilation should last about 1 second and make the chest begin to rise.

NOTE! Minimize interruptions to chest compressions to **less than 10 seconds.**

NOTE! Never attempt more than 2 ventilations before resuming compressions.

Continued

4	The rescuers switch roles about every 2 minutes.

- The rescuer providing compressions calls for a role change by saying "switch" in place of the number "1" in the compression cycle and delivers 30 compressions (for an adult) or 15 compressions (for a child).

- The rescuer providing ventilations delivers 2 ventilations.

- The rescuers switch roles.
  - The rescuer who was providing compressions moves to the person's head, taking their resuscitation mask with them, and prepares to give ventilations by sealing the mask and opening the airway.
  - The rescuer who was providing ventilations moves to the person's side and locates the correct hand position for giving compressions on the chest.

- The rescuer providing compressions begins compressions.

NOTE! Changing positions should take **less than 10 seconds.**

Continued

5	The rescuers continue giving cycles of compressions and ventilations until:	
	• They see signs of ROSC, such as movement, breathing or coughing.	
	• An AED is ready to analyze the heart rhythm.	
	• Other trained providers take over and relieve them from giving compressions and ventilations.	
	• They are too exhausted to continue.	
	• The situation becomes unsafe.	

Skill Sheet 4-4. **CPR—Two Rescuers (Infant)**

NOTE! Complete the rapid assessment and get an AED on the scene as soon as possible.

1	Ensure the infant is on their back on a hard, flat surface. • The rescuer providing compressions stands or kneels to the side of the infant, with their hips at a slight angle. • The rescuer providing ventilations stands or kneels above the infant's head and prepares to give ventilations by sealing the mask and opening the airway to a neutral position.	
2	The rescuer providing compressions gives chest compressions using the encircling thumbs technique. • **Infant:** 15 compressions; compress to a depth of about 1½ inches • Push hard and fast! Give compressions at a rate of 100 to 120 compressions per minute. **NOTE!** Count out loud as you give compressions.	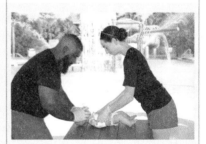

Continued

CPR—Two Rescuers (Infant) (Continued)

3	The rescuer providing ventilations gives 2 ventilations.	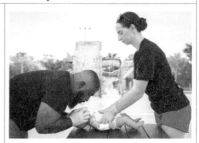

- Give 1 ventilation, pause briefly to allow the infant's chest to fall, then give another ventilation.

- Each ventilation should last about 1 second and make the chest begin to rise.

NOTE! Minimize interruptions to chest compressions to **less than 10 seconds.**

NOTE! Never attempt more than 2 ventilations before resuming compressions.

Continued

4 | The rescuers switch roles about every 2 minutes.

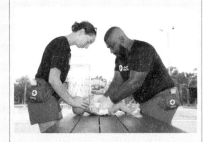

- The rescuer providing compressions calls for a role change by saying "switch" in place of the number "1" in the compression cycle and delivers 15 compressions.

- The rescuer providing ventilations delivers 2 ventilations.

- The rescuers switch roles.
  - The rescuer who was providing compressions moves to the infant's head, taking their resuscitation mask with them, and prepares to give ventilations by sealing the mask and opening the airway.
  - The rescuer who was providing ventilations moves to the infant's side and locates the correct hand position for giving compressions using the encircling thumbs technique.

- The rescuer providing compressions begins compressions.

NOTE! Changing positions should take **less than 10 seconds.**

Continued

5	The rescuers continue giving cycles of compressions and ventilations until:	
	• They see signs of ROSC, such as movement, breathing or coughing.	
	• An AED is ready to analyze the heart rhythm.	
	• Other trained providers take over and relieve them from giving compressions and ventilations.	
	• They are too exhausted to continue.	
	• The situation becomes unsafe.	

Skill Sheet 4-5. **Using an AED**

NOTE! When CPR is in progress, use an AED as soon as one is available. Do not interrupt chest compressions and ventilations until the AED is turned on, the AED pads are applied and the AED is ready to analyze the heart rhythm, unless you are the only rescuer trained to operate the AED and provide CPR.

NOTE! Do not use pediatric AED pads or settings on an adult or on a child older than 8 years or weighing more than 55 pounds (25 kilograms). However, adult AED pads or settings can be used on a child up to 8 years of age or weighing less than 55 pounds (25 kilograms) if pediatric AED pads or settings are not available.

1	Turn on the AED and follow the prompts.	
2	Remove all clothing covering the chest and, if necessary, wipe the chest dry.	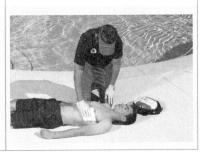

Continued

3	Attach the pads.	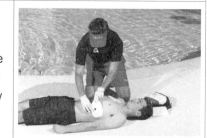
	• Place one pad on the upper right side of the chest and the other on the lower left side of the chest, a few inches below the left armpit.	
	• If the pads may touch, place one pad in the middle of the chest and the other pad on the back, between the shoulder blades.	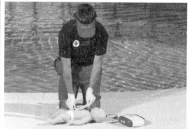
		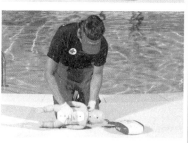
4	Plug the pad connector cable into the AED, if necessary.	

Continued

5	Prepare to let the AED analyze the heart's rhythm.	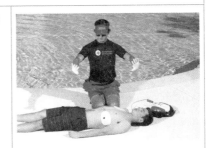

5 Prepare to let the AED analyze the heart's rhythm.

• Make sure no one, including you, is touching the person. Say, "CLEAR!" in a loud, commanding voice.

• If the AED tells you to, push the "analyze" button.

NOTE! When there are two or more rescuers, switch responsibility for compressions each time the AED performs an analysis to limit compressor fatigue. The rescuer responsible for taking over compressions should prepare to resume compressions immediately following the delivery of a shock or after the AED determines that no shock is needed.

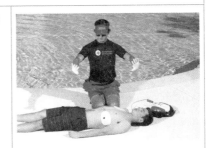

Continued

6	Deliver a shock, if the AED determines one is needed.	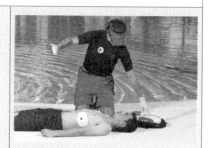
	• Make sure no one, including you, is touching the person. Say, "CLEAR!" in a loud, commanding voice.	
	• Push the "shock" button to deliver the shock.	
7	After the AED delivers the shock, or if no shock is advised, immediately resume CPR, beginning with compressions. Continue giving cycles of compressions and ventilations until:	
	• The AED prompts that it is reanalyzing.	
	• You see signs of ROSC, such as movement, breathing or coughing.	
	• Other trained providers take over and relieve you from giving compressions and ventilations.	
	• You are too exhausted to continue.	
	• The situation becomes unsafe.	

Appendix A
BREATHING AND CARDIAC EMERGENCIES

A:1 ANAPHYLAXIS

Anaphylaxis is a life-threatening allergic reaction that can cause shock and affect the person's ability to breathe. Common allergens associated with anaphylaxis may include venomous insect stings; certain foods (such as peanuts, tree nuts, shellfish, milk, eggs, soy and wheat); medications (such as penicillin and sulfa drugs) and latex.

Recognizing Anaphylaxis

Signs and symptoms of anaphylaxis appear within seconds or minutes of coming into contact with the allergen and may include:

+ Swelling of the face, tongue or lips.

+ Trouble breathing.

+ Signs and symptoms of shock (such as excessive thirst; skin that feels cool or moist and looks pale or bluish; changes in level of consciousness; and a rapid, weak heartbeat).

+ A change in level of consciousness.

To recognize anaphylaxis, look at the situation as well as the person's signs and symptoms (Table 1).

Caring for Anaphylaxis

It is important to act fast when a person is experiencing anaphylaxis, because difficulty breathing and shock are both life-threatening conditions. When you recognize anaphylaxis:

+ Instruct someone to call EMS and get the equipment.

Table 1 Recognizing Anaphylaxis

Situation	Look For:
You do not know if the person has been exposed to an allergen.	• Any skin reaction (such as hives, itchiness or flushing) **OR** • Swelling of the face, neck, tongue or lips **PLUS** • Trouble breathing **OR** • Signs and symptoms of shock
You think the person may have been exposed to an allergen.	Any **two** of the following: • Any skin reaction • Swelling of the face, neck, tongue or lips • Trouble breathing • Signs and symptoms of shock • Nausea, vomiting, cramping or diarrhea
You know that the person has been exposed to an allergen.	• Trouble breathing **OR** • Signs and symptoms of shock

+ If a person is known to have an allergy that could lead to anaphylaxis, they may carry an anaphylaxis kit containing two epinephrine auto-injectors with them at all times. If this is the case, assist the person to use an epinephrine auto-injector (Box 1). A second dose is only necessary if EMS professionals are delayed and the person is still having signs and symptoms of anaphylaxis 5 to 10 minutes after administering the first dose.

+ If the person's healthcare provider has recommended that they carry an antihistamine in their anaphylaxis kit, have the person take the antihistamine according to the medication label and their healthcare provider's instructions. Antihistamines are supplied as pills, capsules or liquids and are taken by mouth. The antihistamine counteracts the effects of histamine, a chemical released by the body during an allergic reaction.

+ Stay with the person and monitor their condition until EMS professionals arrive and begin their care.

Box 1 Anaphylaxis: Assisting with an Epinephrine Auto-Injector

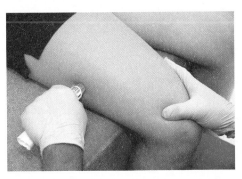

Epinephrine is a drug that slows or stops the effects of anaphylaxis. Epinephrine auto-injector devices, available by prescription only, are syringe systems that administer a single dose of epinephrine by injection. The dose of epinephrine is based on weight (0.15 mg for children weighing between 33 and 66 pounds and 0.30 mg for children and adults weighing more than 66 pounds). Different brands of epinephrine auto-injectors are available, but all work in a similar fashion (and some have audio prompts to guide the user). The device is activated by pushing it against the skin, with the preferred location being the mid-outer thigh. Once activated, the device injects the epinephrine into the thigh muscle. The device must be held in place for the recommended amount of time (about 3 seconds, depending on the device) to deliver the medication. Some medication may still remain in the auto-injector even after the injection is complete. After removing the auto-injector, you may need to massage the injection site for several seconds, depending on the device. Follow the manufacturer's instructions.

When you recognize anaphylaxis, if the person carries an epinephrine auto-injector with them, assist the person to use it as needed. If the person is unable to self-administer their medication, you may administer the medication to them, if it is allowable by state laws and regulations and you are trained and authorized to do so. Where state laws and regulations allow, some facilities keep a stock

Continued

Box 1 Anaphylaxis: Assisting with an Epinephrine Auto-Injector (Continued)

epinephrine auto-injector for designated staff members who have received the proper training to use it in an anaphylaxis emergency. If you are using a stock epinephrine auto-injector, follow your facility's protocols, which may include verifying that the person is showing signs and symptoms of anaphylaxis, ensuring that the person has been prescribed epinephrine in the past and making sure to use a device containing the correct dose based on the person's weight.

To administer epinephrine to a person using an epinephrine auto-injector, obtain consent and follow these general guidelines.

1. Verify the medication with the person. Check the label for the medication name and expiration date.

2. Remove the cap and any safety device on the auto-injector.

3. Locate the outside middle of one thigh to use as the injection site.

4. With one hand, hold the person's leg firmly to limit movement while you administer the medication. With the other hand, quickly and firmly push the auto-injector tip into the person's thigh at a 90-degree angle. It is OK to do this through clothing, if necessary.

5. Hold the auto-injector in place for 3 seconds after a click is heard.

6. Massage the injection area for 10 seconds, if indicated by the device manufacturer's instructions.

7. Note the time of administration and any change in the person's condition. Administer a second dose only if EMS professionals are delayed and the person is still having signs and symptoms of anaphylaxis 5 to 10 minutes after administering the first dose.

8. Dispose of the auto-injector in a sharps container, or give it to EMS professionals for disposal.

Additional training on administering epinephrine for anaphylaxis is available through the American Red Cross, if you need it.

A:2 ASTHMA ATTACK

Asthma is a chronic illness in which certain substances or conditions, called triggers, cause inflammation and narrowing of the airways, making breathing difficult. Common triggers include exercise, temperature extremes, allergies, respiratory infections, stress or anxiety, air pollution and strong odors. Exposure to the trigger causes narrowing of the airways and increased mucus production, making it harder for the person to breathe and resulting in what is known as an "asthma attack."

Even when a person takes steps to manage their asthma by avoiding triggers and taking prescribed long-term control medications, they may still experience asthma attacks occasionally. Many people who have been diagnosed with asthma have an asthma action plan (a written plan that the person develops with their healthcare provider that details daily management of the condition as well as how to handle an asthma attack).

Recognizing an Asthma Attack

Signs and symptoms of an asthma attack include:

+ Wheezing or coughing.
+ Rapid, shallow breathing.
+ Trouble breathing.
+ A feeling of tightness in the chest or a feeling of being unable to get enough air into the lungs.
+ An inability to talk without stopping for a breath in between every few words.
+ A change in cry or a weak cry (in infants and young children).
+ A limited ability to walk or climb stairs.
+ Anxiety and fear.
+ Fatigue.
+ Sweating.

Caring for an Asthma Attack

An asthma attack can become life-threatening because it affects the person's ability to breathe. If a person has signs and symptoms of an asthma attack:

+ Instruct someone to call EMS and get the equipment.

+ Assist the person to follow their asthma action plan, if they have one. This may include using a prescribed quick-relief (rescue) medication for the emergency treatment of an asthma attack. Encourage the person to use their prescribed quick-relief medication, assisting as needed (Box 2). More than one dose of medication may be needed to stop the asthma attack. The medication may be repeated after 10 to 15 minutes.

+ Stay with the person and monitor their condition until they are able to breathe normally or EMS professionals arrive and begin their care.

Box 2 Asthma: Assisting with Quick-Relief (Rescue) Medications

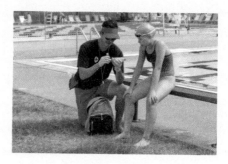

Quick-relief (rescue) medications are taken when the person is experiencing an acute asthma attack. These medications work quickly to relax the muscles that tighten around the airways, opening the airways right away so that the person can breathe more easily. These medications are often given through a metered dose inhaler, which delivers a measured dose of the medication directly into the person's lungs. A spacer (or chamber) may be used to make it easier for the person to coordinate their breathing with the inhaler so that they receive the full dose of medication. The medication enters the spacer, and then the person inhales the medication through the mouthpiece on the spacer. For infants and young children, a spacer may be used with a face mask instead of a mouthpiece.

When you recognize that a person is having an asthma attack, encourage them to use their prescribed quick-relief medication,

Continued

Box 2 Asthma: Assisting with Quick-Relief (Rescue) Medications (Continued)

assisting if needed. If the person is unable to self administer their medication, you may administer the medication to them, if it is allowable by state laws and regulations and you are trained and authorized to do so. To administer quick-relief medication to a person using a metered dose inhaler, obtain consent and follow these general guidelines.

1. Verify the medication with the person. Check the label for the medication name and expiration date. Use only the medication prescribed for the person, and verify that it is for the quick relief of an acute asthma attack.

2. Shake the inhaler and remove the mouthpiece cover.

3. Attach the spacer (and the face mask, if necessary) to the inhaler.

4. Tell the person to breathe out as much as possible through the mouth.

5. Have the person place their lips tightly around the mouthpiece (or place the face mask over the person's nose and mouth).

6. Administer the medication.
   + **If the person uses a spacer:** Firmly press the inhaler canister to release the medication into the spacer. Tell the person to take a slow, deep breath and then to hold their breath for 5 to 10 seconds. If the person cannot take a slow, deep breath or they are using a spacer with a face mask, tell them to take several normal breaths from the spacer.
   + **If the person does not use a spacer:** Have them take a long, slow breath (about 3 to 5 seconds) while pressing down on the top of the inhaler canister. Then have the person hold their breath for 5 to 10 seconds.

7. Note the time of administration and any change in the person's condition. The medication may be repeated after 10 to 15 minutes.

Additional training on administering quick-relief medications for asthma is available through the American Red Cross, if you need it.

A:3 HEART ATTACK

A **heart attack** occurs when blood flow to part of the heart muscle is blocked. Because the cells in the affected area of the heart muscle are not receiving the oxygen and nutrients they need, they become damaged and can die. The damage can affect the heart's ability to pump normally, and in some cases, may lead to cardiac arrest. Activating the EMS system as soon as you recognize the signs and symptoms of a heart attack can minimize the damage to the heart and may save the person's life.

Recognizing a Heart Attack

Signs and symptoms of a heart attack include:

+ Chest discomfort or pain, which can range from mild to unbearable. The person may complain of pressure, squeezing, tightness, aching or heaviness in the chest. The pain or discomfort is persistent and usually lasts longer than 3 to 5 minutes, or it may go away and then come back. It is not relieved by resting, changing position or taking medication. It may be difficult to distinguish the pain of a heart attack from the pain of indigestion, heartburn or a muscle spasm.

+ Isolated or unexplained discomfort or pain that spreads to one or both arms, the back, the shoulder, the neck, the jaw or the upper part of the stomach.

+ Dizziness or light-headedness.

+ Trouble breathing, including noisy breathing, shortness of breath or breathing that is faster than normal.

+ Nausea or vomiting.

+ Pale, ashen (gray) or slightly bluish skin.

+ Sweating.

+ A feeling of anxiety or impending doom.

+ Extreme fatigue.

+ Unresponsiveness.

Although men often have the "classic" signs and symptoms of a heart attack, such as chest pain that radiates down one arm, women may have more subtle signs and symptoms or experience the signs and symptoms of a heart attack differently than men do. For example, in women, the "classic" signs and symptoms may be milder or accompanied by more general signs and symptoms, such as back pain, shortness of breath, nausea or vomiting, extreme fatigue, or dizziness or lightheadedness. Because these signs and symptoms are so general and nonspecific, women may experience them for hours, days or even weeks leading up to the heart attack but dismiss them as nothing out of the ordinary. The signs and symptoms of a heart attack may also be more subtle in people with certain medical conditions, such as diabetes.

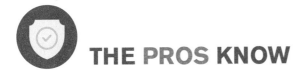

THE PROS KNOW

Most people who die of a heart attack die within 2 hours of first experiencing signs or symptoms. If you suspect a heart attack, always respond as if the person is experiencing one, and activate the EMS system immediately.

Caring for a Heart Attack

If you think that a person is having a heart attack:

+ Instruct someone to call EMS and get the equipment.

+ Have the person stop any activity and rest in a comfortable position. Loosen any tight or uncomfortable clothing. Reassure the person. Anxiety increases the person's discomfort.

+ Offer aspirin if the person is awake, can follow simple commands, can chew and swallow, and is allowed to have aspirin. Aspirin helps prevent blood clots from forming and is most effective when given soon after the onset of signs and symptoms of a heart attack. Before offering aspirin, ask the person, "Are you allergic to aspirin?" and "Have you ever been told by a healthcare provider to avoid taking aspirin?" If the person answers "no" to each of these questions, you can assist them with taking two to four low-dose (81-mg) aspirin tablets (162 to 324 mg) or one regular-strength (325-mg) aspirin tablet. Have the person chew the aspirin completely. Never delay calling EMS or getting equipment to find or offer aspirin. Also, do not offer the person an aspirin-containing combination product meant to relieve multiple conditions or non-aspirin pain medications, such as acetaminophen (Tylenol®), ibuprofen (Motrin®, Advil®) or naproxen (Aleve®). These medications do not work the same way aspirin does and are not beneficial for a person experiencing a heart attack.

+ If the person has a history of heart disease and takes a prescribed medication to relieve chest pain (for example, nitroglycerin), offer to assist with the medication.

+ Closely monitor the person's condition until EMS professionals arrive and begin their care of the person.

+ Be prepared to perform CPR and use an AED.

A:4 OPIOID OVERDOSE

Opioids are drugs that are prescribed to reduce pain. Misuse of, and addiction to, these prescription drugs has increased the frequency of opioid overdose–related deaths in the United States. In addition, use of non-prescription illegal forms of opioids, such as heroin, also contributes to opioid overdose–related deaths.

Examples of prescription opioids include hydrocodone (Vicodin®), oxycodone (OxyContin®, Percocet®), oxymorphone (Opana®), codeine (used alone or in combination with Tylenol® or cough medicine), morphine (Kadian®, Avinza®), and fentanyl. Street names for illegal non-prescription forms of opioids (heroin) include Brown Sugar, China White, Dope, H, Horse, Junk, Skag, Skunk and Smack.

Recognizing Opioid Overdose

Opioid overdose suppresses the drive to breathe and can quickly lead to respiratory failure, respiratory arrest or cardiac arrest. Signs and symptoms of opioid overdose include:

+ The presence of items associated with drug use (such as prescription pill bottles, pipes, needles, syringes or pill powder).

+ Decreased breathing effort (for example, breathing slowly and perhaps only a few times per minute).

+ Gasping or gurgling.

+ Bluish or grayish skin.

+ A decreased level of consciousness or unresponsiveness.

+ Pinpoint pupils (pupils that are abnormally small under normal lighting conditions).

Caring for Opioid Overdose

When you recognize signs and symptoms of an opioid overdose:

+ Instruct someone to call EMS and get the equipment.

+ Provide care for the conditions found and consider naloxone (Box 3).

  – If the person is in respiratory failure or respiratory arrest, give ventilations and administer naloxone as soon as it is available and resources permit. You may also administer emergency oxygen, if it is available and you are trained to do so.

  – If the person is in cardiac arrest, prioritize high-quality CPR and use of an AED. Administer naloxone when it is available and resources permit, but do not delay or pause CPR or use of an AED to do so.

  – If the person is responsive but has a decreased level of consciousness, or if the person is unresponsive but has a pulse and is breathing normally, consider naloxone if you know or suspect that opioid overdose is the cause.

+ Stay with the person and give care as you have been trained until EMS professionals arrive and begin their care. Have the person rest comfortably, monitor their condition and provide reassurance.

Box 3 Opioid Overdose: Assisting with Naloxone

Naloxone (Narcan®), a drug that temporarily reverses the effects of opioids, is given through the nose using a nasal atomizer or nasal spray. You may administer naloxone that is stocked at your facility, if allowable by state laws and regulations and you are trained and authorized to do so. Under some state laws and regulations, you may also administer naloxone that is prescribed to the person.

To administer naloxone to a person using a nasal spray device, obtain consent and follow these general guidelines.

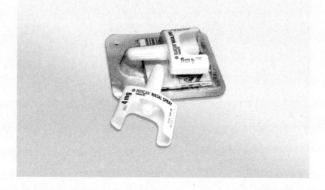

1. Check the label for the medication name and expiration date.

2. Hold the device with your thumb on the bottom of the plunger and two fingers on either side of the nozzle.

3. Place and hold the tip of the nozzle in either nostril until your fingers touch the bottom of the person's nose.

4. Press the plunger firmly to release the dose into the person's nose.

Continued

Box 3 Opioid Overdose: Assisting with Naloxone (Continued)

To administer naloxone to a person using a nasal atomizer, obtain consent and follow these general guidelines.

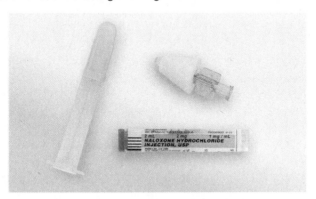

1. Check the label for the medication name and expiration date.
2. Uncap the naloxone medication vial and the syringe or uncap the prefilled syringe.
3. Attach the medication vial to the syringe, if necessary.
4. Screw the nasal atomizer onto the top of the syringe.
5. Split the dose between both nostrils. Place the nasal atomizer in the person's nostril. Push firmly on the medication vial to release about half of the medication into the nostril. Repeat with the other nostril.

Note the time the naloxone was administered and look for changes in the person's condition. If the person is still having signs and symptoms 2 to 3 minutes after administering the first dose of naloxone and EMS professionals have not arrived, administer a second dose, using a new nasal device. Monitor the person until EMS professionals arrive and begin their care.

Additional training on administering naloxone for opioid overdose is available through the American Red Cross, if you need it.

GLOSSARY

Abandonment: the withdrawal of support or help from another person, despite having the responsibility to provide this support or help

Abdominal thrusts: inward and upward thrusts just above the navel; used in combination with back blows to force the object out of the airway when an adult or child is choking

Agonal breaths: isolated or infrequent gasping in the absence of normal breathing

Airway: the pathway from the mouth and nose to the lungs

Anaphylaxis: a severe, life-threatening allergic reaction

Aspiration: inhalation of foreign matter, such as saliva or vomit, into the lungs

Assessment: the process of gathering data about the emergency and the person to help determine next actions

Asthma: a chronic illness in which certain substances or conditions (triggers) cause inflammation and narrowing of the airways, making breathing difficult

Back blows: blows between the shoulder blades, used in combination with abdominal thrusts or chest thrusts to force the object out of the airway when a person is choking

Bag-valve-mask (BVM) resuscitator: a hand-held device used by two rescuers to give ventilations to a person in respiratory or cardiac arrest

Basic airway: a device that is inserted through a person's mouth or nose to keep the airway clear and provide a channel for air movement and suctioning

Bloodborne pathogen: a disease-causing microorganism that is spread when blood from an infected person enters the bloodstream of a person who is not infected

Cardiac arrest: a condition in which the heart has stopped beating or is beating too ineffectively to circulate blood to the brain and other vital organs

Chest compression fraction (CCF): an indicator of CPR quality; represents the percentage of time during the resuscitation effort spent performing chest compressions

Chest thrusts: quick thrusts into the center of a person's chest used to force the object out of the airway when a person is choking

Consent: permission to give care

Direct transmission: a method of passing a pathogen from one person to another; the pathogen is passed through physical contact or droplet spread

Emergency medical services (EMS) system: a network of professionals linked together to provide the best care for people in all types of emergencies

Frothing: white or pinkish foam or froth around the nose and mouth following a drowning; caused by a mix of mucus, air and water during respiration

Gas exchange: the molecular process of adding oxygen to, and removing carbon dioxide from, the blood

Heart attack: a condition that occurs when blood flow to part of the heart muscle is blocked, causing cells in the affected area of the heart muscle to die

Hypoxia: low oxygen levels in the body's tissues

Implied consent: permission to give care that is not expressly granted by the person but is assumed because circumstances exist that would lead a reasonable person to believe that the person would give consent if they were able to

Indirect transmission: a method of passing a pathogen from one person to another; the pathogen is passed by way of a contaminated surface or object or by a vector

Level of consciousness: a person's state of awareness, alertness and wakefulness

Nasopharyngeal airway (NPA): a type of basic airway that is inserted through the nose and extends to the back of the throat

Negligence: the failure to do what a reasonable and careful person would be expected to do in a given situation

Occupational exposure: contact with blood, body fluids or other potentially infectious materials that may occur while a person is performing their job duties

Occupational Safety and Health Administration (OSHA) Bloodborne Pathogens Standard: a federal regulation that specifies measures employers are required to adhere to in order to protect employees from exposure to bloodborne pathogens while on the job

Oropharyngeal airway (OPA): a type of basic airway that is inserted through the mouth and fits over the tongue to hold it up and away from the back of the throat

Pathogen: harmful microorganisms that can cause disease

Personal protective equipment (PPE): a barrier device that is worn or used to prevent pathogens from contaminating the skin, mucous membranes or clothing and lower the risk for getting or transmitting an infectious disease

Professional rescuer: paid or volunteer personnel who have a legal duty to act in an emergency

Recovery position: a side-lying position used to lower a person's risk for choking and aspiration when the person is unresponsive but breathing, or responsive but not fully awake

Respiration: the process of moving oxygen and carbon dioxide between the atmosphere and the body's cells; includes ventilation and gas exchange

Respiratory arrest: absence of breathing

Respiratory failure: a condition that results when ventilation is not sufficient to sustain gas exchange; as a result, the blood contains too little oxygen, too much carbon dioxide, or both

Resuscitation mask: a transparent, flexible device that fits over a person's mouth and nose and is used to give ventilations without making mouth-to-mouth contact or inhaling exhaled air

Return of spontaneous circulation (ROSC): successful resuscitation, evidenced by the return of a regular heart rhythm capable of sustaining adequate blood flow throughout the body

Scope of practice: the range of tasks a professional rescuer is legally allowed to do

Shout-tap-shout sequence: technique used to check for responsiveness

Sign: an indicator of injury or illness that another person can observe

Single-rescuer CPR: cardiopulmonary resuscitation in which one rescuer transitions between giving sets of chest compressions and ventilations

Standard precautions: infection control practices that are used to prevent the transmission of pathogens that are carried in blood, body fluids or other potentially infectious materials; they should be followed at all times and with every person

Stoma: a surgically created opening in the neck

Sudden cardiac arrest: cardiac arrest that happens suddenly and without any warning signs or symptoms

Symptom: an indicator of injury or illness that only the injured or ill person can report

Two-rescuer CPR: cardiopulmonary resuscitation in which one rescuer gives chest compressions and the other gives ventilations

Vector: an insect or animal, such as a mosquito, tick or rodent, that carries and transmits a pathogen

Ventilation: the mechanical process of moving air into and out of the body

Ventricular fibrillation (V-fib): an abnormal heart rhythm in which the heart muscle simply quivers (fibrillates) weakly instead of contracting strongly so that there is no circulation

Ventricular tachycardia (V-tach): an abnormal heart rhythm in which the heart muscle contracts too fast for effective circulation

REFERENCES

American Red Cross. (2011, 2016, 2021). *First aid/CPR/AED.*

American Red Cross. (2011, 2017). *Emergency medical response.* The StayWell Company, LLC.

American Red Cross. (2012, 2016). *CPR/AED for professional rescuers.*

American Red Cross. (2012, 2016). *Lifeguarding.*

American Red Cross. (2017). *Responding to emergencies: Comprehensive first aid/CPR/AED.* The StayWell Company, LLC.

American Red Cross. (2021). *American Red Cross focused updates and guidelines.* https://www.redcrosslearningcenter.org/s/sac-2021-focused-updates-guidelines

American Red Cross Scientific Advisory Council, Aquatics Subcouncil. (2021). *CPR for drowning.* https://www.redcrosslearningcenter.org/s/science

American Red Cross Scientific Advisory Council, First Aid Subcouncil. (2016). *Gloves for first aid.* https://www.redcrosslearningcenter.org/s/science

American Red Cross Scientific Advisory Council, First Aid Subcouncil. (2019). *Hand hygiene.* https://www.redcrosslearningcenter.org/s/science

American Red Cross Scientific Advisory Council, Resuscitation Subcouncil. (2020). *Naloxone timing of re-dosing.* https://www.redcrosslearningcenter.org/s/science

American Red Cross Scientific Advisory Council, Resuscitation Subcouncil. (2020). *Opioid toxicity recognition by laypersons.* https://www.redcrosslearningcenter.org/s/science

Centers for Disease Control and Prevention. (2022, June 30). *About HIV.* U.S. Department of Health and Human Services. https://www.cdc.gov/hiv/basics/whatishiv.html

Centers for Disease Control and Prevention. (2021, May 20). *AIDS and opportunistic infections.* U.S. Department of Health and Human Services. https://www.cdc.gov/hiv/basics/livingwithhiv/opportunisticinfections.html

Centers for Disease Control and Prevention. (2021, April 21). *Body fluids that transmit HIV.* U.S. Department of Health and Human Services. https://www.cdc.gov/hiv/basics/hiv-transmission/body-fluids.html

Centers for Disease Control and Prevention. (2018, June 18). *Standard precautions: Summary of infection prevention practices in dental settings.* U.S. Department of Health and Human Services. https://www.cdc.gov/oralhealth/infectioncontrol/summary-infection-prevention-practices/standard-precautions.html

Centers for Disease Control and Prevention. (2022, March 30). *Viral hepatitis: Hepatitis B: Frequently asked questions for health professionals.* U.S. Department of Health and Human Services. https://www.cdc.gov/hepatitis/hbv/hbvfaq.htm#treatment

Centers for Disease Control and Prevention. (2020, August 7). *Viral hepatitis: Hepatitis C questions and answers for health professionals.* U.S. Department of Health and Human Services. https://www.cdc.gov/hepatitis/hcv/hcvfaq.htm#b1

National Institute for Occupational Safety and Health. (1989, February). *A curriculum guide for public safety and emergency response workers: Prevention of transmission of acquired immunodeficiency virus and hepatitis B virus* (Publication No. 89-108). U.S. Department of

Health and Human Services, Public Health Service, Centers for Disease Control. https://www.cdc.gov/niosh/docs/89-108/default.html

Occupational Safety and Health Administration. (2011, January). *OSHA fact sheet: OSHA's bloodborne pathogens standard*. https://www.osha.gov/sites/default/files/publications/bbfact01.pdf

Occupational Safety and Health Administration. (n.d.). *Bloodborne pathogens and needlestick prevention*. U.S. Department of Labor. Retrieved April 7, 2023 from https://www.osha.gov/bloodborne-pathogens/hazards.

STOCK PHOTOGRAPHY CREDITS

Chapter 3

Page 70   shutterstock.com/
           TomoTaro

Chapter 4

Page 263   Shutterstock.com/curtis

Appendix A

Page 160   shutterstock.com/Bob
           LoCicero

INDEX

in respiratory failure, 32, 52–54, 158, 159, 164
suctioning in, 50, 55, 60–61, 89–90
ventilations given in, 12, 31–33, 48–49, 53–59, 80–88
Breathing techniques. *See* Ventilations

C

Cardiac arrest, 32, 105
Cardiac emergencies, 149–150
   AED use in, 104, 106–110, 119–129, 145–148
   cardiac arrest, 32, 105
   cardiopulmonary resuscitation (CPR) in, 109–119
   chain of survival in, 105–107
   heart attack, 156, 157
   oxygen in, 62–70, 93
Cardiopulmonary resuscitation (CPR)
   in adults, 117–118
   airway opening in, 23, 28–29, 31–33 43–44, 47–50
   barriers for personal protection in, 9–12, 17, 19, 164
   chest compressions in. *See* Chest compressions
   in children and infants, 107, 117–118
   multiple rescuers, 99, 103, 127–129
   one rescuer, 59, 109–111, 118, 127–128, 164
   two rescuers, 59, 124, 128, 137–144, 164
   ventilations in. *See* Ventilations
Chain of infection, 7–8
Chest compressions
   in airway obstruction, 51, 54, 71, 95, 100
   in cycle with ventilations, 109, 111, 116–118, 128–129, 133, 136, 139–140, 143–144, 148
   effectiveness of, 111, 113, 129–130
   in multiple-rescuer response, 127–129
   in one-rescuer CPR, 118
   in two-rescuer CPR, 111–112, 119
Chest thrusts for obstructed airway, 72–74, 76–77, 95, 98, 102, 163
Children
   AED use on, 108–109, 122–123, 145–148

bag-valve-mask resuscitators for, 58
chest compressions in, 110–112, 116–118, 124, 127, 130–131, 134, 137
resuscitation masks for, 57
two-rescuer CPR in, 111–112, 118
ventilations in, 12, 23, 31–33, 48–50, 53, 55–56, 61, 76, 77, 78, 80–88, 116, 118, 136, 139, 143
Choking, 71–278. *See also* Airway Obstruction
Circulation
   in cardiac emergencies, 149
   pulse checks of, 30–31
Clothes drag, 41
Consent to care, 6, 19, 27, 34, 72, 163–164
   implied, 6, 27, 72, 96, 100

D

Defibrillation, 106
Direct transmission of disease, 8, 14–15
   in pool water, 7
Droplet transmission of disease, 8
Duty to act, 4

E

Emergency medical services (EMS)
   in cardiac chain of survival, 105–107
   in heart attack, 156–157, 163
   when to activate, 35–36
Encircling thumbs technique, 115
Engineering controls, bloodborne pathogens, 14, 16–17
Epinephrine, 151–152

F

Fibrillation, 120
   ventricular, 119–120, 165
Frothing, 32, 60, 163

G

Gloves, 10–11, 13, 20–21, 126
Gowns, as personal protective equipment, 10–11

H

Hand hygiene for infection control, 9
Head-tilt/chin-lift maneuver, 28, 43, 53,
    56, 80, 116
Heart attack, 156–157, 163
Hepatitis B, 14–15, 17
    risk of transmission, 14–15
    vaccination against, 17
Hepatitis C, 14–15
    risk of transmission, 14–15
High-efficiency particulate air (HEPA)
    filter, 10, 12
HIV infection and AIDs, 14
Hypoxia, 51, 63, 70, 163

I

Implied consent, 6, 164
Indirect transmission of disease, 8,
    14–15, 164
Infants
    AED use on, 109, 122–123, 145
    age range of, 108
    airway obstruction in, 51, 54, 71,
        95, 100
    bag-valve-mask resuscitators for,
        58–59
    chest compressions in, 77, 109–112,
        116–118, 124, 130–131, 134
    oxygen therapy in, 67–68
    pulse check in, 30
    resuscitation masks for, 57, 80
    two-rescuer CPR in, 118, 119
    ventilations in, 31–32, 48, 50, 53,
        54–55, 56–57, 80–88, 110,
        111, 117
Infections
    from bloodborne pathogens, 11

J

Jaw-thrust maneuver, 29, 43–44, 47, 53,
    82, 85
    with head extension, 29, 43–44, 47,
        53, 55, 82, 116
    modified, 29, 44, 47, 53, 55, 85, 116

L

Legal considerations, 3–6, 27, 38, 96, 100

M

Masks
    nonrebreather, 68–70, 93
    as personal protective equipment,
        10–12
    resuscitation. See Resuscitation masks
Mask-to-stoma ventilations, 55–56, 164
Metal surfaces, and AED use, 125
Mouth-to-mouth ventilations, 56
Mouth-to-nose ventilations, 56
Moving a person
    clothes drag, 41
    two-person seat carry, 41
    walking assist, 41
Multiple rescuers
    in cardiac emergencies, 63, 149
Myocardial infarction, 105

N

Nasal cannula, 67, 68
    oxygen delivery with, 32, 63–64,
        66–70, 79, 94
Nasopharyngeal airway, 61–62, 164
Needlestick injuries, 14–15, 18
Negligence, 4, 164
    and Good Samaritan laws, 5
9-1-1 calls, 3
Nitroglycerin transdermal patch, AED
    use in, 126
Nonrebreather mask, 68–70, 93
    oxygen delivery with, 32, 63–64,
        66–68, 70, 79, 94

O

Occupational Safety and Health
    Administration (OSHA), 16, 164
Opportunistic infections, 14–15, 167
Oropharyngeal airway, 61–62, 164
Oximetry, pulse, 70–71
Oxygen, 31–32, 50–52, 56–59, 62–71,
    79, 91–94, 119, 125
    cylinders, 64–66
    delivery devices, 67–68, 70, 79
    fixed-flow-rate, 63, 69–70
    safety precautions with, 64–65
    saturation monitoring, 70–71
    variable-flow-rate, 63, 91–94

in head, neck and spinal injuries, 55, 87

mask-to-stoma, 55–56

in multiple-rescuer CPR, 99, 103, 127–129

in one-rescuer CPR, 118

with resuscitation mask. *See* Resuscitation masks

in two-rescuer CPR, 39, 111–112, 118–119, 165

Ventricular fibrillation, 120, 165

Ventricular tachycardia, 120, 165

Viruses, 12, 14

  HIV, 14–16, 36, 150, 167

personal protective equipment in exposure to, 9–12, 17, 19, 164

risk of transmission, 12, 14–15

vaccination against, 14, 17

Vomiting, 15, 35, 53, 150, 156–157

W

Walking assist, 41

Wet conditions, AED use in, 122, 125–126

Wheezing, 37, 153

Work practice controls, 17